A Guide to the Methodologies of Homeopathy

Further copies of this book and other titles may be ordered at
www.cuttingedgepublications.co.uk

All enquiries should be addressed to
mail@cuttingedgepublications.co.uk

First published in 1991. This revised edition published in 2004 by
Cutting Edge Publications
PO Box 156
Totnes
Devon
TQ9 6ZP
England

A catalogue record for this book is
available from the British Library

ISBNB 0 9517657 6 0

Foreign translations of this book are available - for current details visit:
http://www.ianwatsonseminars.com/moxie/read/books

Original Cover illustration: David Tomkins
Original typesetting: Paul Wood

A Guide to the Methodologies of Homeopathy

by Ian Watson

Revised Edition

Cutting Edge Publications
Totnes
Devon
England

By the Same Author

Books
Aspects of Homeopathy - Musculo-skeletal Problems
Cutting Edge Publications 2004 ISBN 0 9517657 4 4
The Tao of Homeopathy
Cutting Edge Publications 2004 ISBN 0 9517657 2 8

Recorded Seminars in Audiotape and Digital CD Format
A Remedy for Everything!
A Remedy for Everything Else!
Casetaking and Case Analysis
Dynamic Homeopathy
Dynamic Materia Medica
Health and the Planets
Homeopathy and the Chakras
Mental and Emotional Health
Musculo-Skeletal Problems
Organ Remedies
Seven Herbs: Indications and uses of Herbal Tinctures
Skin Problems: Healing from Within
The Natural Traveller
Therapeutics and Layers
Understanding the Miasms

More information and online ordering available at
www.ianwatsonseminars.com

Trade discounts available to all retailers and educational establishments

Contents

Acknowledgements

I am indebted to Robert Davidson for creating the context within which this book could be written. I would also like to thank Robin Murphy N.D. for teaching with such clarity, and Kenneth Metson for demonstrating to me how simple the appropriate use of homeopathy really is. Thanks are due also to Susan Barber for her help with the text, to Paul Wood for his technical skill and personal support and to Sally for never doubting that I would get it finished. I am also particularly grateful to my patients for continuously demanding of *me* the flexibility of mind that I continuously preach to others.

We teach best what we most need to learn ....

Ian Watson
Sparkbridge,
Cumbria
1990

Introduction

An average group of doctors eavesdropping on a conversation amongst an average group of homeopaths have much in common with a martian who accidentally picks up the cricket commentary. One of my goals for homeopathy is that it may be picked up and used by anyone in a way that is more or less commensurate with their current level of understanding and expertise.

By way of example, anyone who knows what a bruise is should know how and when to use *Arnica*. All those trained in first aid procedures should also know when to use *Aconite, Hypericum, Rhus tox., Opium, Ruta, Symphytum* and a few others. Midwives should know all of this, and also when to use *Caulophyllum, Ipecac., Sabina, Pulsatilla* and others relevant to their art. Surgeons should find no difficulty in applying the virtues of *Bellis perennis, Calendula, Staphysagria* and *Strontium carb.* And so on.

Prevalent amongst many of the current teachers and practitioners of homeopathy is a desire to teach homeopathy at its highest (and most difficult) level. Whilst I share this desire, my belief is that adhering to this goal *exclusively* is a positive hindrance to the widespread development of homeopathy. The majority of those who could be using homeopathy right away are deterred or prevented from doing so by the formidable effort and shifts in understanding that seem to be required.

It is with this in mind that I have written this book. My hope is that anyone with an interest in homeopathy and a familiarity with its basic principles will be stimulated to learn one or more of its many applications and, more importantly, to *use* what they have learnt in the healing of the sick.

All of the methods described herein have proven their worth by achieving curative results for those who have used them. I have included as little as possible that is not supported by my own experience, as the existing homeopathic literature already contains an excess of second-hand material.

The major purpose of this book then, is to expose the reader to a wide cross-section of the many diverse ways in which the principle of *similars* may be applied in practice. My intention is not to produce confusion in those for whom homeopathy is a simple and straightforward affair. Rather I would hope that practitioners and students at all levels will feel encouraged to widen the scope of their prescribing beyond their own and, hopefully my own, present limitations.

Foreword to the Revised Edition

It hardly seems possible that thirteen years have passed and more than ten thousand copies have been sold since this book first came into being.With no advertising except personal recommendation it has continued to sell steadily both in the U.K. and overseas, and I would like to thank all of those who have recommended the book to friends and colleagues over the years.

The primary motivation behind producing a revised edition was my embarassment at the fact that I was still, through the pages of this book, advocating the use of Kent's repertory! It was, as many will remember, the only half-decent repertory around ten years ago, but since then we have been blessed with a profusion of superior products. I still encounter students struggling to get to grips with Kent's old classic from time to time, and it has troubled me no end to think that I was inadvertantly recommending it. This new edition, then, is my attempt to put the record straight and, as far as is possible in a book of this size, to introduce the reader to a few further 'methodologies' that I have encountered in recent years.

I have done little to alter the original text, simply updating here and there and occasionally adding a few comments. I was surprised to realise how much of the original text did, in my view, seem to stand the test of time. The main revision takes the form of several completely new chapters which I have inserted alphabetically amongst the original ones.

Some Further Acknowledgments

A word of thanks is due to all those who have taken the trouble to write to me over the years with feedback and encouragement. Thanks are also due to my colleagues and friends at *The Lakeland College* who have tolerated my frequent absences and changes of direction with good humour and loving support. In particular I would like to acknowledge Anne Waters for being so consistently supportive. I am also grateful to all of the students and practitioners that I have met on my travels who have been willing to share the journey with me. Finally, I would like to thank Ken Teppin for assisting me and supporting my work in many different ways, including pestering me to finish this revised edition.

Ian Watson
Devon
2004

It is possible to obtain the needed correspondence in a great variety of ways and degrees, and one practitioner will find it in one way and another in another.

J. H. Clarke
Dictionary of Practical Materia Medica

Abbreviations used in the text

b.d.	twice daily
t.d.s.	three times daily
q.d.	four times daily
p.r.n.	as required
h.	hour (e.g. 2h = every 2 hours)
s.d.	single dose
c.s.d.	collective single dose
dps	drops
Ø	mother tincture
ext.	externally

Aetiologies

By far the most frequent excitement of the slumbering psora into chronic disease, and the most frequent aggravation of chronic ailments already existing, are caused by grief and vexation.

Samuel Hahnemann
Chronic Diseases

Definition
ætiology = 'the assignment of a cause'.
A prescription is based primarily on some past trauma, illness or event rather than on the presenting symptoms. The stronger the cause-and-effect relationship between the trauma and the presenting state, the more an ætiological prescription is indicated.

Direct Aetiology
In cases with a direct ætiology there is a clear and direct relationship between the presenting problem and the trauma which preceeded it, no matter how long the problem has persisted. For example, when a patient says "I have had recurrent headaches ever since a head injury three years ago", that is a direct ætiology. In such a case I would be looking for a "head injury" remedy first, using the symptoms of the case to differentiate between the remedies in that group (*Arn., Nat-s., Cic.* etc.). Kent's repertory[1] contains many ætiological rubrics showing those remedies which, from clinical experience, we know have an established reputation in curing ailments following a particular trauma, be it grief, fright, bad news, vaccination, injury, poisoning etc. The appropriate rubric is a good starting place in a case displaying a direct ætiology.

Sometimes when the cause and effect relationship is very clear, particularly if there are no outstanding symptoms in the case, the ætiology can completely over-rule symptomatology as the basis for the prescription. Thus it is that our 'trauma' remedies such as *Aconite, Arnica* and *Hypericum* have cured many symptoms and conditions which never appeared in their respective provings.

How to Prescribe
In a case having a direct ætiology there are three choices for the prescriber. The prescription may be based on the ætiology alone, on the symptoms alone or on a combination of the two. I find that wherever possible the third option is the most reliable one, but the ætiology should be used as a starting point provided there are remedies known to have that ætiology as a confirmed indication.

If the remedy is prescribed only on the symptoms of a case and the ætiology isn't covered, that remedy may well cure but often it will only palliate. A remedy which covers the ætiology but not the symptoms of the case will generally cure dramatically or do nothing at all. A cure is most likely to result if the remedy covers the ætiology *and* bears similarity to the symptoms of the case.

To illustrate the above, imagine a case of convulsions following head injury.

The symptoms of the case are:

Convulsions   epileptiform
                   worse from excitement
                   worse from being touched
                   with opisthotonos

A remedy which covers this case symptomatically would be *Belladonna*, but *Belladonna* is not known to have cured conditons brought about by injury to the head. Whilst it may well ameliorate the symptoms, it may or may not bring about a lasting cure. A remedy which covers the ætiology but not the symptoms would be *Arnica;* again this remedy may or may not cure. If the ætiology of 'Head injury, ailments after' is taken as the starting point, the remedies to be considered would be: *Arnica, Cicuta, Hypericum, Natrum mur.*, and *Natrum sulph*. Of these, the one which bears greatest similarity to the symptoms is *Cicuta,* and that remedy would have a greater likelihood of being curative than the other two.

Prescriptions based on a direct ætiology are often best given in a single dose of a medium or high potency (30th upwards) as the response is usually clear and obvious if the remedy acts curatively. If low potencies are preferred for any reason these will also prove curative in ætiological cases, but the remedy may need to be repeated frequently over a period of time.

Case examples
A woman complained of flu-like symptoms which had persisted for four days. She had a dull, frontal headache; nausea and loss of appetite; general lethargy; aching limbs. All of these symptoms are common to many remedies and to many flu-like conditions, hence are of limited prescribing value. I enquired about the onset of the complaint and discovered that the symptoms had appeared within several hours after the patient had been involved in a minor car accident, in which she was shaken but unhurt physically. Ignoring

2

the symptoms, I prescribed *Aconite* 200 on the direct ætiology 'Ailments from fright', and she reported that everything cleared up within a few hours.

Sometimes a direct ætiology will simplify cases that may otherwise prove difficult to treat. An example I saw was a woman in her mid-fifties with a small breast tumour which had been diagnosed as cancerous. She was naturally in a state of great anxiety and was due to have surgery in a few week's time. On taking her case I found her general health to be good and she was constitutionally very strong. I discovered that the tumour had been preceeded by an injury to the breast, which had been badly bruised. As the bruising slowly subsided, the lump made its appearance right on the site of the injury. With such a clear ætiology, in a person of previous good health, I felt there was a good prognosis under homeopathic treatment.

As far as I could determine from the literature there are only two remedies known to have cured tumours following injury to the breast - *Bellis perennis* and *Conium*. Being unable to differentiate them on the symptoms present, I proceeded to give *Bellis* 6 t.d.s. for a fortnight. After a few days treatment she developed intolerable itching on her hands, face and eyes, so she stopped taking the remedy. The itching quickly disappeared, but the lump was absolutely unchanged.

My interpretation was that this was a partial proving of *Bellis*, as no curative result was obtained and the itching was not a return of an old symptom. Given that there were only a few days left before the date of the operation, I decided to play my only remaining card and give her *Conium*. A look in my remedy kit revealed *Conium* 6 and *Conium* CM - these were the only two potencies I had available! Seeing that we had little to lose and she was virtually resigned to having the surgery, I gave a dose of the CM with bated breath. The result was that when she went to have the operation a few days afterwards the tumour couldn't be found, much to her embarassment, the surgeon's disappointment, and my delight!

Hidden or Suppressed Aetiology
In some cases there existed at one time a clear cause and effect relationship between trauma and disease-image, but owing to the passage of time or as a result of suppressive treatment, that relationship has become obscured. These may present as difficult cases which either do not display a clear prescribing image, or where symptomatically-indicated remedies only palliate. In such a case it may be necessary to trace the origin of the problem carefully to see if there is a hidden ætiology that has been overlooked. If such is found, a

3

prescription based on the ætiology and the symptoms *which used to be present* may be the curative remedy.

Case Examples

One of the best examples of this method is found under the *Mezereum* picture in Tyler's *Homeopathic Drug Pictures*[2] . Here she relates a case of deafness cured by Carroll Dunham with *Mezereum* 30, the prescription being based on a skin eruption that had been totally suppressed years previously, and of which no trace was apparent. Ignoring the deafness, which had no distinguishing symptoms, Dunham obtained details of the skin eruption that had preceded it and found the remedy most similar to those original symptoms, even though they were now completely hidden. *Mezereum* was prescribed retrospectively and proved to be the curative remedy.

Another favourite case of mine which is worth studying in this regard is related by Dr. Allen in his *Materia Medica of The Nosodes*[3] . This is a case of impotence which Dr. Wesselhoeft had failed to cure with his best prescriptions. Finally, the patient visited the great Adolph Lippe, who's careful questioning revealed that the man had suffered diphtheria ten years previously which had been allopathically treated, and he had never fully recovered. The nature of the diphtheria attack was that it went from one side of the throat to the other, then back to the original site. On this keynote and the fact that the diphtheria attack seemed to have directely preceded the man's troubles, Lippe prescribed *Laccaninum* CM and cured the patient, impotence and all.

I treated an eight year old girl suffering with headaches, catarrh, adenoids and partial deafness. Symptomatic and miasmatically indicated remedies produced little response, so I questioned more closely about traumas in the past. It transpired that the girl had been concussed as a baby, had broken her arm in a fall three years previously, had fallen and injured her face one year ago and had recently tumbled down an entire flight of stairs, banging her head on the way. On this basis I prescribed a single dose of *Arnica* 10M which resulted in a complete cure of all the symptoms, and she became less liable to fly off the handle as well. I have also used *Arnica* successfully in children of various ages where there was a history of a physically traumatic birth, particularly a forceps delivery, when indicated remedies had failed to act.

Indirect Aetiology

There are two main types of indirect ætiology. The first is where a person has been in a certain environment, family dynamic or any other life or work situation which has, *over a period of time*, lowered that person's level of health and has contributed to their becoming sick. For example, a sensitive child who was bullied occasionally at school, was afraid to tell anyone, gradually lost his self-confidence, and now suffers with timidity and a fear of new situations. If the presenting state had resulted directly from a single incident, then it would be a direct ætiology, perhaps 'ailments from fright' or 'ailments from mortification'. The cause and effect relationship is not that clear however, so the presenting symptoms would be a more reliable guide to the prescription in this case, taking into account the circumstances which have been contributory.

The second type is where a person had an illness or possibly an operation at some time which lowered their general state of health, although they may appear to have fully recovered. As a result of this they become susceptible to new problems which start to manifest over a period of weeks or months.

For example, I treated a woman who had glandular fever in her teens from which she seemed to recover. Gradually however, over a period of many months, she became far more susceptible to colds and influenza, each bout leaving her a little more debilitated than the previous one. The following year, the colds started to settle on her chest and she suffered bronchitis three times in succession. The point to take note of is that the problems she presented with did not *directly* result from the glandular fever. Rather the original illness left a residual weakness which eventually manifested in new health problems.

In cases where there is an indirect ætiology, usually there is a lapse of time before any new problems start to manifest, whereas direct ætiologies tend to produce a much more rapid and obvious alteration in health. With indirect ætiologies, the presenting symptoms should always take precedence over the original stress for purposes of prescribing, but the stressful situation, if known, will often help to confirm the remedy picture. Often in constitutional prescribing, the circumstances and events of childhood, taken collectively, will help to confirm the indicated remedy. As an example, many adult patients who require *Aurum* constitutionally are found to have been pressured to succeed by their parents, or were forever trying to keep up with an elder sibling who was the apple of their parents' eye.

Multiple Aetiologies
Chronic cases often contain multiple ætioligies in the history, each of which has added something to the picture that finally presents itself for treatment. It is helpful for understanding and treating these cases if a timeline is drawn showing the chronological sequence of events (see Layers).

Where a specific drug or toxin has created the presenting image, and an indicated remedy cannot be found or fails to cure, a tautopathic prescription is often of great benefit (see Tautopathy). Where a specific illness has left a never-been-well-since situation, this can be said to be an acquired miasm (see Miasms).

One of my favourite cases in the entire homeopathic literature illustrates beautifully the use of multiple ætiologies as a basis for the prescription. It was originally submitted to *The Homeopathic World* in 1924, and is reprinted in Clarke's *Prescriber*[4] on pages 55-58. I am not going to retell the tale here but would hope that the reader will be tempted to seek out the reference and study the case closely.

Repertory Updates
When a remedy prescribed on the basis of symptom-similarity cures a condition dating from a particular trauma, it is important that it be added to the appropriate rubric in the repertory if it is not already there. For example, I have seen *Antimonium tartaricum* cure several pathological states in children which arose following vaccination, and now have this remedy added to my repertory under the rubric 'Vaccination, ailments after'.

We should also be creating new ætiological rubrics relevant to the stresses and traumas peculiar to our twentieth century lifestyle. One such example which I have entered in my repertory is 'Contraceptive pill, ailments after'. This rubric contains *Arnica, Folliculinum, Natrum mur., Pulsatilla* and *Sepia,* all of which I have verified clinically in this situation, and I am sure other remedies could be added.

Ideally we should have a clinical database to which any practitioner may contribute and from which everyone would benefit enormously, otherwise most of the invaluable clinical wisdom relevant to our age will disappear for ever.

Further Reading

Dr. Eswara Das & Dr. Radha
Synopsis of Homeopathic Ætiology - A Complete Work on Causation
World Homeopathic Links, New Delhi-110055, India

D. M. Foubister
Tutorials in Homeopathy
Beaconsfield Publishers, Beaconsfield, England

Dr. P. Sankaran
The Importance of Ætiology in Homeopathy (A Symposium)
Homeopathic Medical Publishers, Santa Cruz, Bombay

Arborivital Medicine

Definition

This method takes its name from the words *arbor* (tree) and *vita* (life). It was introduced by R.T. Cooper (1844-1903) and involves prescribing single-drop doses of plant mother tinctures, which have preferably been prepared from fresh living specimens.

As far as I am aware, this method fell into neglect and is not in use today, but some of the results obtained by Cooper, and later by his son Dr. Le Hunte Cooper suggest that it is worthy of re-investigation.

Background

The arborivital method is based on Cooper's hypothesis that a curative action is an inherent property of all living plants, and that this does not require trituration, succussion or dilution to be released. In his booklet *Cancer and Cancer Symptoms[1]* he wrote: "I found that there existed in plant remedies a force which Hahnemann had strangely left unacknowledged, and which acted by virtue of a power in all respects similar to a germinating power in the human body."

Cooper drew analogy between the growth force evident in plants and the similar force which manifests in the growth of a tumour in the human body. Both to him represented a latent power which required suitable soil in which to produce growth. His method of treatment consisted of bringing together in the body two corresponding forces and this, he found, produced curative results. This is undoubtedly an ingenious application of the law of similars!

Preparation & Use

Whilst Cooper wrote that ordinary homeopathic mother tinctures could be utilised, it was his experience that tinctures made in a different way were even more effective when administered in single-drop doses.

He developed a simple method of preparation which involves taking a living plant, in full bloom wherever possible, and immersing a flowering stem, together with some leaves, lightly crushed between the fingers, into a clear vial containing proof spirit. If possible, the vial is then placed in direct sunlight and left there until the colour is leached from the plant material - up to an hour is usually sufficient. Whether exposed to sunlight or not, the plant material is then removed, the vial is corked and the remedy is ready to use.

Sometimes he would prepare tinctures by immersing a shoot or twig in alcohol whilst it was still attached to the plant or tree, and he considered this to be a superior method of extracting the latent curative properties. Remedies which were made in this way and then exposed to sunlight he termed 'heliosthens'.

Cooper was insistent that the remedies be administered in a single dose which must be allowed to act fully before any repetition. He would generally dispense the remedies in the form of a powder medicated with a single drop of the tincture, this to be taken dry on the tongue on an empty stomach. Having administered a dose, he would meticulously record any reaction to the remedy, whether in the form of cured clinical symptoms, aggravations or proving symptoms brought out in those particularly sensitive. This accumulated data helped him to put together clinical pictures of numerous remedies about which little or nothing was previously known, many of which are recorded in Clarke's three-volume *Dictionary of Practical Materia Medica*, identified by the initials R.T.C.

Indications for Prescribing

Quite from where Cooper obtained his indications is a mystery in many cases, but it is known that he relied heavily on observation of natural phenomena and took many leads from the *Doctrine of Signatures*. For example, it is recorded[2] that Dr. Skinner mentioned to him that *Hydrangea* was a useful remedy for diabetes. Cooper consulted a botanical work which described *Hydrangea* as 'the thirstiest shrub known', which he related back to Dr. Skinner as confirmation of his clinical tip. The observation that marigolds close their petals in cloudy weather led him to prescribe *Calendula* successfully in cases of deafness and other complaints which were aggravated in cloudy or overcast weather. He also noted that "aggravation from damp" was a leading indication for *Lemna minor*, a plant which flourishes in ponds. Those accustomed to lateral thinking will find the homeopathic materia medica becomes a rich field of study when approached in this way. However, the more logically minded can prescribe remedies in arborivital form based on ordinary symptom-similarity and good results will still be obtained.

When to Use the Method

Cooper claimed that arborivital remedies were most appropriately used in cases which were incurable by other means, traditional homeopathic methods included. The two categories of disease to which he devoted particular attention were cancer and chronic deafness, and he obtained remarkable curative results in both areas.

9

His comments on the treatment of cancer are particularly pertinent, where his experiences led him to write: "............the most easily acted upon of all forms of chronic disease are the tumours, especially internal ones, whether cancerous or otherwise......... The matter, then, is one of sympathetic relationship: the life of a collection of cancer cells obeys the same laws as the life of any other material body. It has come into being by a process of germination and is to be dispersed by a force that sets agoing a similar but antagonising process.

The difficulty of cure lies in the difficulty of discovering the sympathetic force. But just as the experienced gardener knows the conditions that are most favourable for development of the energies of certain seeds, so ought the experienced practitioner to know the conditions that in the diseased patient will call into activity the curative energies of his remedy.

.........it will suffice to say that I have met with very little difficulty in this particular class of diseases in arriving at the indicated remedies[3] ."

I have prepared my own tinctures of *Bellis perennis, Agraphis nutans, Taraxacum, Hypericum perfoliatum* and several others by the arborivital method but have insufficient experience in using them to draw any firm conclusions. It is my hope that interest in the arborivital method will be rekindled in the future and it will take its deserved place in the homeopath's toolkit.

Case Example
The following case is extracted from an article submitted by Cooper to *The Homeopathic World[4]* in 1899.

"A lady brought her twenty year-old daughter to me, suffering with hydrocephalus since infancy, but recently becoming worse. Her head measured 27.5 inches in circumference and there were two large oedematous swellings on the nape of the neck. Being interested at the time in the action of our common ivy, and having conluded that it possessed a special relationship to certain phases of rickets, I placed an arborivital drop of *Hedera helix* upon her tongue.

The result was almost amazing. The next morning a clear fluid began dripping away from her nostrils, and continued to drip for three weeks, and simultaneously the two oedematous swellings at the back of her neck began to reduce in size, until with the cessation of the discharge they completely disappeared. The discharge was so great as to necessitate the use of twenty to thirty pocket handkerchiefs a day. Along with this the size of the head went down, and when, thirteen months after, the young lady was measured for a new hat it was found that the circumference of her head was now 25 inches.

I repeated the dose of *Hedera* once when the symptoms of brain pressure seemed to be returning. This second dose proved completely effectual, and since then the girl's entire disposition has changed, and from being nervous, unhappy and diffident she has become lively, cheerful and active. The circumference of the head remains at 25 inches, but in no other way is inconvenience felt."

Further Reading

R.T. Cooper
Cancer and Cancer Symptoms
Jain Publishing Co., New Delhi, India

Constitutional Prescribing

Ten years of practice will be a revelation to you, so that you will understand people and their minds. You will almost know what they are thinking, and will often take in a patient's constitution at first glance.

James Tyler Kent
Lesser Writings

Synonyms: Kentian homeopathy; Classical homeopathy; Centralist prescribing; Essence prescribing

Definition

Simply stated, it involves taking the whole person into account as far as this is possible, and treating the person simultaneously on all levels - physical, mental and emotional. The expression 'treat the person, not the disease' may be more accurately applied to this method than to any other.

Under this heading are included many different ways of prescribing all of which share the common thread of treating the whole rather than the parts, the patient rather than the disease. In this chapter the type of constitutional homeopathy which has gained prevalence in recent years and which seems especially suited to the current age will be discussed. This I have chosen to call 'psychosomatic prescribing'.

The other major constitutional approach, which is far less widely practised today than formerly, emphasises the physical general symptoms above all else, and this I have treated separately under the heading 'Physical Generals'.

Introduction

Constitutional prescribing is the cornerstone of any successful homeopathic practice. At the same time, this method is undoubtedly the most difficult and the most challenging of all, particularly for the inexperienced practitioner. Probably the majority of those who attempt to master it fail to do so, even after years of study. Constitutional prescribing is nonetheless the most attractive if not seductive of all the techniques available, for several reasons. Firstly, the results obtainable can often appear both to practitioner and patient to be bordering on the miraculous. Secondly, the method allows an incredible degree of individual artistry to be brought into play without detracting from the results. And finally, the emphasis on the psychological components of remedies and patients is very much in keeping with the cultural trend of recent years, such that it blends in beautifully with many of the prevalent spiritual and psychological models.

Psychosomatic Prescribing
In *The Organon*, paragraphs 210-213, Hahnemann drew attention to the importance of the mental and emotional state of the patient when seeking to find the curative remedy. It fell to J. T. Kent (1849-1916) to explore this area of homeopathy in depth and to develop it into a system of prescribing in its own right. To accomplish this Kent blended his vast homeopathic expertise with his study of the teachings of the Swedish mystic Emmanuel Swedenborg.

The resulting 'Kentian' method operates from a philosophical standpoint in which disease is seen to flow from the innermost regions of a human being to the outermost. In other words, a person is perceived to be dis-eased on a spiritual or mental/emotional level first, and this imbalance pervades the immaterial vital body (the 'simple substance'), which finally produces changes ('ultimates') on the physical level. Therefore in order to cure disease, treatment has to proceed in the same direction, the prescription being aimed towards the innermost mental and emotional state rather than the outward physical expression. Within the confines of this model, it is considered that to prescribe upon the local symptoms of disease or the physical organs will result in a suppression, that is to say it will be detrimental to the patient as a whole.

Hierarchy of Symptoms
When the case has been fully taken, those symptoms which are considered to be characteristic (see Symptoms chapter) are graded in importance in the following hierarchical order:

First   Mental and emotional symptoms (Kent considered the symptoms pertaining to the will, that is the emotions to be the most important; those of the understanding or intellect to be next most important and those pertaining to the memory to be of lesser importance)

Second Physical general symptoms (those pertaining to the whole person e.g. chilliness, fever, sweat, sleep, sexual function, menses, food cravings & aversions etc.)

Third   Physical particulars & disease symptoms (those pertaining to certain parts of the organism or to the disease state itself e.g. headache, arthritis, chilblains, coryza etc.)

Wherever possible, the remedy prescribed must bear similarity to the mental/ emotional state, as this is perceived as being fundamentally causative. In the absence of clear mental/emotional symptoms, the physical general symptoms are given precedence. Disease symptoms and local symptoms are considered the end results of disorder on the higher levels, and are therefore given the lowest hierarchical importance.

Kent's *Repertory* is the most widely used tool in constitutional prescribing, the mind section being particularly indispensable despite the fact that the language used is neither simple nor everyday. Once the structure of the repertory has been understood it can be used with great flexibility to guide the prescriber towards the indicated remedy.

Prescribing method
The prescribing rules to be applied in this method are very clearly defined and it is intrinsic to the method that certain of them must be strictly adhered to. The actual prescribing method evolved from Hahnemann's directions in the fifth edition of *The Organon.*

The prescription should take the form of a single remedy, in a single dose, in a predominantly high potency (generally within the range 30 - CM). A key component is the necessity to then wait until the response to the prescription has clearly ceased before repeating or re-prescribing. (Whilst Hahnemann later abandoned this rule in favour of frequently repeated doses, it remains standard practice in constitutional prescribing to this day. This is almost entirely due to the influence of Kent's teachings which were based on the fifth edition of *The Organon,* the sixth edition having been withheld from publication until 1921, five years after Kent's death. In this final edition Hahnemann directed that the medicine should be repeated every day, and was by this time using the new 50-millesimal potency scale in favour of the centesimal potencies).

If and when a repetitition of the same remedy is indicated, it may either be given in the same potency as before, or in the next highest potency, according to Kent's (centesimal) potency scale as follows:

30 - 200 - M - 10M - 50M - CM - DM - MM

The format followed by most practitioners is to prescribe in the above manner and to assess the response to the prescription at intervals of a month or longer. Often very subtle changes are seen to take place over a prolonged period of time, hence the need for relatively infrequent follow-ups. It is not uncommon for a patient to be given no further medicine for many months after the original dose. It is therefore frequently necessary to do much explaining to patients, particularly those new to homeopathy who are accustomed to taking their medicine on a rather more regular basis. Not surprisingly, many practitioners will give placebos during the waiting period to satisfy their patient's expectations.

Several variants on the theme of a 'single dose' have been developed and are widely used. These include a *split dose* (two doses of the same potency at intervals of 4-12 hours); a *collective single dose* (three doses of the same potency at intervals of 4-24 hours) and an *ascending collective single dose* (three doses in ascending potencies at intervals of 4-24 hours, e.g. 30-200-1M or 200-1M-10M). These deviations are employed to ensure that the remedy has 'taken hold' and, in the case of the latter, to minimise aggravation, which in my experience it appears to do. Anyone who doubts this should give *Natrum mur.* 200 to a series of patients in whom the remedy is well-indicated and note how many of them develop a headache soon after taking it! A similar number of patients given *Natrum mur.* 30-200-1M will be found to benefit from the remedy without suffering a headache. Insufficient evidence, perhaps, but it suggests to me that combining potencies in this way does produce a different reaction which may be of advantage to the patient.

Case examples
Often in psychosomatic prescribing the behaviour, moods, gestures and language of the patient are of paramount importance and these symptoms must be carefully perceived and interpreted into the language of the repertory and materia medica if a successful prescription is to be made.

Case One
A seven year old boy was brought to me with what was described as a phobia, the problem being that he had an aversion to eating except when he was at home. He wouldn't eat at school, nor in cafes and restaurants, and when I asked him why this was he said he was worried that he might be sick. Several years ago he had been sick all night and that had worried him a lot.

His only physical problem was a persistent cough, sneezing bouts and a blocked nose. He would often wake with a blocked nose and it would remain blocked even after blowing.

I enquired some more about his character and behaviour and he volunteered that when he was drawing he always liked it to be perfect. He said: "nearly everything I draw I go wrong on; but I get it right eventually." His mother said he seemed to spend a lot of time folding up his clothes, and he always liked his hair to be just right. She also remarked that he liked his trainers to be nice and clean, which they were.

In the context of a boy of his age, I felt that his *fastidiousness* was the most characteristic feature of the case, and of the remedies known to be fastidious *Arsenicum album* has more concern with cleanliness and tidiness than any other. On this basis I gave him a single dose of *Arsenicum* 1M.

The subsequent report was that the day after he took the remedy he ate everything at school for the first time, and had not been concerned about eating out since. His respiratory symptoms had completely disappeared and his mother felt he had generally been a lot calmer. She also remarked that he had stopped pulling out his eyelashes, something which he had done for years but she had forgotten to mention at the first visit.

He remained well for about two months after the initial dose, when the remedy was repeated in the same potency in response to a return of several of the symptoms.

Case Two
A fifty-four year old woman presented with low energy, sore eyes and recurrent colds. She had a tendency to constipation; cold hands and feet; weak ankles; waking unrefreshed; a blistering eruption on the backs of her hands. She had a fear of being shut in, e.g. in lifts; she had always been very independent and had never married. She was quite closed and rarely displayed her feelings. All of her symptoms were on a functional level only, and these combined with her personality type clearly indicated *Natrum muriaticum*, which was given in 30-200-1M.

I saw her a month later and she reported improvement in every respect. This she found astonishing as her father had died the day after she took the remedy, which was naturally upsetting. I took this to be a case of synchronicity, given that *Natrum mur.* is a major remedy for the effects of grief. She continued in good health for one and a half years without any further medicine, when a partial return of her symptoms called for a repeat of *Natrum mur.*, which was given in a single dose of the 10M potency with continued improvement.

Natrum mur. is such a frequently indicated remedy, it seems that one could run a whole practice prescribing little else, at least here in Britain. It is one of those polychrest remedies that even a novice prescriber can learn to spot very quickly.

Case Three
A woman in her forties complained of depression for many years and a tendency to frequent headaches. The depression manifested sometimes as irritability and anger, triggered off by little things. The patient said: "I get cross very easily. I don't like to be criticised. I wish I wasn't like this. It's not fair on the family to have to put up with me." At other times she would become introverted and low in her spirits: "I never want to join in with anything, I have no enthusiasm for life. I shouldn't be like that, should I? I think it's wrong of me." She went on to describe how she felt during one of the headaches: "I felt awful. All I wanted to do was die. It would have been so easy to take a bottle of aspirin. Every time I opened my eyes I saw a big black hole and just wanted to die."

In this case the *language* of the patient gave a clear guide to her internal state. One is reminded often of Hahnemann's injunction to record the symptoms in the *patient's own words* rather than interpreting or translating them. Using Kent's *Repertory*, I chose the following rubrics to represent the patient's symptoms:

Reproaches herself (page 71)
Despair with the pains (page 35)
Suicidal from pains (page 85)

It is interesting that in this case there was nothing about the nature of the headaches that was particularly unusual, but how they affected her emotionally was highly characteristic and therefore had to be present in the remedy. I am sure that most readers will recognise *Aurum metallicum* in the above picture, which was given in the 1M and later the 10M potencies with complete relief of both the headaches and the depression.

Use of Low Potencies
Kent repeats frequently in his writings[1] that a homeopath should know when to use the whole range of potencies from the tincture to CM and above, but the majority of his published cases contain only high potency prescriptions. Probably as a result of this, most constitutional prescriptions today are made using medium to high potencies exclusively.

Whilst these guidelines have served and continue to serve many practitioners adequately in a majority of cases, I have many times applied the constitutional approach to a case, but prescribed a low potency (6c or 12c) in repeated doses, varying the frequency to suit the individual. I find this variation achieves very satisfactory results, and is particularly suitable in cases where there is a likelihood of the treatment being antidoted, for instance by drugs or coffee, or where aggravation needs to be minimised. The beauty of giving repeated doses is that the worst the patient can do is to antidote the effects of one or two doses, which makes little difference to the overall response, whereas if a single dose is given that means the entire treatment could potentially be wiped out by a single cup of coffee.

Case examples
I treated a man suffering intermittent deafness and tinnitus in this way, the prescription being *Aurum metallicum*, based primarily on his mental state which was one of violent anger and intolerance of contradiction, together with a history of heart trouble. So as to reduce the probability of aggravation I gave *Aurum* 6 t.d.s., under which his hearing problems, general energy, mental state and (so he told me) his golf swing all improved! He took the remedy for several months on a daily basis and suffered no aggravation or ill-effect.

I have found that acute hay fever will often dissappear with the indicated constitutional remedy, in cases where remedies prescribed only on the hay fever symptoms such as *Allium cepa* have failed to work or have only palliated. I saw a girl who had suffered for weeks with very severe symptoms. Her eyes were red raw from rubbing, she was sneezing almost non-stop and was in a generally pitiful state. The interesting thing was that she came into my consulting room, complained of feeling too hot and promptly fainted! On this indication together with her mild nature and strong desire for consolation I gave her *Pulsatilla* 12 every 4 hours and she was transformed within two days. She reduced the frequency to one dose every few days and remained symptom-free for the remainder of the summer.

Further Developments
Whilst the Kentian method can only truly be said to have been practised by Kent, many have been sufficiently influenced by his teachings to base the bulk of their practising style on his teachings. In the past, these have included Herbert A. Roberts, Margaret Tyler, Marjorie Blackie, and more recently Elizabeth Wright-Hubbard, Pierre Schmidt and Pablo Paschero. Major developments have been made by the Greek homeopaths George Vithoulkas and Vassilis Ghegas, and also Catherine Coulter, Ananda Zaren, Alize Timmerman and many others throughout the world who have all extended and refined the work on personality profiles of remedies begun by Kent. The

level of refinement to which this area of homeopathy has been taken in recent years is quite remarkable.

Another contemporary worker in this field was the late Edward Whitmont, who added his own experience and insight to the psychological profiles of the polychrest remedies. Other contributors include Rajan Sankaran, Joseph Reeves and Eugene Candegabe who have each developed their own variations on the Kentian theme of a 'central disturbance' out of which all else flows, and their respective teachings have gained wide acceptance in recent years, particularly amongst European and American homeopaths.

When to Prescribe Constitutionally
In Great Britain and the United States the Kentian method is now so widely taught and practised that many are misled into believing that it is the *only* way to practise homeopathy. If the existence of other methods is acknowledged, the Kentian method is often elevated by its proponents to the status of *pure homeopathy*, *classical homeopathy* or even *Hahnemannian homeopathy* (!). This need by some to be seen as the sole bearers of truth has, in my opinion, created greater disagreement and division amongst homeopaths than anything else.

The constitutional approach is most appropriate in chronic *functional* disorders, where there are well-marked mental/emotional and general symptoms. This would embrace a wide spectrum of patients with disorders such as allergies, digestive problems, insomnia, migraines, menstrual and menopausal disturbances, behavioural and emotional disorders etc., etc. Any problem that may be defined as psychosomatic in origin (i.e. the disorder originates in the mind or psyche) will generally be found very suitable for this type of treatment, as will the inumerable 'syndromes' for which no organic cause can be found.

The constitutional method is generally less appropriate in advanced & serious degenerative pathologies, also in heavily drugged & (allopathically) suppressed cases. Although good results can still be obtained with constitutional prescribing in these types of cases, a very high level of skill is required and often a change of technique will produce a more gratifying outcome. I myself have struggled unsuccessfully for months to unravel complex cases with constitutional prescriptions, when a subsequent change of approach has rendered the case far easier to manage and put the patient on the long road back to health. Unfortunately many prescribers feel that they are letting the patient (or themselves, or homeopathy) down by abandoning the constitutional approach in favour of another, possibly more appropriate, technique. I find that provided the interests and wishes of the patient are kept predominantly in mind, such self-reproach will be unnecessary.

Drawbacks
There are several drawbacks to the constitutional approach that are worth mentioning. The first is that the curative response to a single dose of a high potency remedy can sometimes be quite fragile and susceptible to being easily antidoted by substances such as coffee, toothpaste and drugs, to name but a few. It has been stated that even subtle factors such as taking the remedy whilst exposed to direct sunlight can cause it to be antidoted! This means that a co-operative and self-disciplined patient is required, which excludes a fair proportion of the population. As I have mentioned already, this problem can often be overcome by the use of a low potency prescription administered in repeated doses.

The second drawback is that the case-taking and subsequent analysis can be very time-consuming and, as has already been mentioned, it requires a very high level of skill and perception on the part of the prescriber in order to achieve consistently successful results. This puts homeopathy out of the reach of many would-be practitioners, and especially there are large numbers of doctors who are dissuaded from using homeopathy at all in their practices, largely because they see the constitutional method as being so difficult and requiring such an enormous investment of time. I am sure that if doctors (for instance) were first taught how to use some of the other methods of homeopathy effectively, particularly the therapeutics and organ-based methods, they would be much more able to incorporate these into their practices and, with further experience, would find it a natural progression to gradually learn the constitutional approach.

A third drawback is that where constitutional prescriptions are based primarily on the mental/emotional state of the patient, this effectively limits the number of remedies that are available for use to those whose psychological profiles have been well-defined. Whilst this number is ever-increasing, it still represents a very small proportion of our vast homeopathic materia medica, and a great deal of work in this area remains to be done.

Within the limitations mentioned, constitutional homeopathy presents a wonderful on-going challenge to every homeopath, and the rewards are extremely gratifying once a level of proficiency has been attained.

Further Reading

P. Bailey
Homeopathic Psychology
North Atlantic Books, Berkeley, California 94704, U.S.A.

M. Blackie
Classical Homeopathy
Beaconsfield Publishers Ltd., Beaconsfield, Bucks.

E. Candegabe
Comparative Materia Medica
Beaconsfield Publishers Ltd., Beaconsfield, Bucks.

C. R. Coulter
Portraits of Homeopathic Medicines, Vols 1-3
North Atlantic Books, Berkeley, California 94704, U.S.A.

D. Gibson
Studies of Homeopathic Remedies
Beaconsfield Publishers Ltd., Beaconsfield, Bucks.

J. T. Kent
Lectures on Homeopathic Philosophy
Lectures on Materia Medica
Lesser Writings
Jain Publishing Co., New Delhi-110055, India

H. A. Roberts
The Principles and Art of Cure by Homeopathy
Jain Publishing Co., New Delhi, India

R. Sankaran
The soul of Remedies
Jain Publishing Co., New Delhi-110055, India

M. L. Tyler
Homeopathic Drug Pictures
C.W. Daniel Co., Ltd., Saffron Walden, Essex

G. Vithoulkas
The Science of Homeopathy
Grove Press Inc., New York
Essence of Materia Medica
Jain Publishing Co., New Delhi, India

E. Wright-Hubbard
Homeopathy as Art and Science
Beaconsfield Publishers, Beaconsfield, England

Genus Epidemicus

Definition

A prescription is based on Hahnemann's[1] observation that during a true epidemic of acute disease a majority of cases will respond to the same remedy, provided the remedy is similar to the characteristic symptoms of the epidemic.

Prescribing technique

Details are taken of the characteristic symptoms (see *Symptoms*) of a number of cases during the epidemic, and these are put together to form an image of the disease in its entirety. A remedy is chosen which bears greatest similarity to the characteristics of this complete image, and if it is found to act curatively in the majority of cases it may be said to be the genus epidemicus of that epidemic. Such a remedy will also act prophylactically for contacts who have not yet developed symptoms of the disease.

When to Use the Method

This method appears to be most applicable to the more serious acute diseases such as cholera, typhoid, smallpox etc., although this is not exclusively the case. The homeopathic literature suggests that the acute diseases of childhood such as measles and whooping cough could be effectively treated by this means where a number of cases are found to occur in the same locality. Epidemic influenza is another area where the method could be successfully employed. I have yet to find opportunity to employ this method in my own practise.

Case Examples

Certain remedies have found fame through being used successfully in epidemic outbreaks. Reisig of New York found *Lac caninum* to be the genus epidemicus for an outbreak of malignant diphtheria[2], and the astounding results he obtained caused the remedy to be accepted by those who had previously scorned the idea of using potentised bitch's milk as a medicine. It is recorded[3] that Hahnemann recommended the administration of *Cuprum*, *Veratrum* or *Camphor*, according to the symptoms of the case, for the sufferers of a cholera epidemic. This was despite the fact that he had not seen any of the patients for himself but had studied carefully the case reports sent by others. His suggestions, when acted upon proved remarkably effective nonetheless. Tyler reminisces[4] how *Pyrogen* was found to be the genus epidemicus for every single case of an influenza epidemic she was called to treat.

Further Reading

D. Shepherd
Homeopathy in Epidemic Diseases
Health Science Press, Saffron Walden, Essex

R. P. Mathur
Common Infectious Diseases with Therapeutics and Repertory
Jain Publishing Co., New Delhi, India

S. Hahnemann
Organon of Medicine 6th Edition, paras. 100-103
Jain Publishing Co., New Delhi, India

R. P. Mathur
Common Infectious Diseases with Therapeutics and Repertory
Jain Publishing Co., New Delhi, India

Group Analysis

Definition
This refers to the method of thematic prescribing developed by Jan Scholten and his colleagues in Holland and elsewhere. The method involves identifying the key themes which relate to the minerals and elements, enabling these to be matched to similar themes in patients. The result is that whole groups of remedies, such as the *Calciums* and *Ferrums*, may be studied together, and remedy differentiation and selection is made considerably easier.
See also: Thematic Prescribing

Introduction
It was Kent, I believe, who put forward the idea that if we were to prove just one kingdom of nature thoroughly then we would have a fairly complete materia medica. Given the diversity within the plant and animal kingdoms, the minerals and elements are the only kingdom that can readily be explored in this way. In his *Lesser Writings*, Kent included a number of remedy pictures that were created by combining what he already knew about the constituent components of some of the polychrest mineral remedies. For example, from his knowledge of *Silica* and the potassium salts such as *Kali-carb.* and *Kali-bich.*, he was able to assemble a fairly detailed picture of *Kali-silicatum*. By replacing the *Silica* component with *Arsenicum*, he pieced together a tentative picture of *Kali-arsenicosum*, and by substituting *Alumina* in place of potassium, he arrived at a picture of *Alumina-silicate*. Thus was a new way of expanding the materia medica created!

In 1993 Jan Scholten's book *Homeopathy and Minerals* was first published in English, giving a detailed description of the key themes belonging to many of the major minerals and elements used in homeopathy. This enabled many of the gaps to be filled in with regard to the materia medica of the mineral kingdom, expanding the pictures of familiar but not so well-known remedies, and introducing a number of completely new remedies at the same time. I, like many others, was both intrigued and a little overwhelmed at the possibilities that Scholten opened up.

The emphasis of Scholten's work was to develop the psychological themes of the elements, and this led him to reveal a number of insights which seemed incredible in their simplicity and precision. For example, he claimed that the *Carbonicums*, as a group, all had issues with the father, whilst the *Muriaticums* all had mother issues. That idea alone gave me enough food for thought for many months! Eventually, after some deliberation, I decided that the only way to test the validity of his claims was to try some of the remedies based on the pictures he described. As was my habit, I ordered in a supply of some of the strange new combinations and awaited my chance to try them out. I didn't have to wait very long.....

Case Examples
One of my first cases where I was able to apply the group analysis method to good effect was a woman who had back trouble, a tendency to weight gain, periodic headaches and a history of suppressed grief. Her overall appearance and the physical generals of the case pointed strongly towards *Calc.-carb.* as the indicated remedy, yet her emotional state of suppressed grief, inability to cry and with a tendency to periodic headaches suggested *Natrum-mur.*.

My usual strategy in a case like this would have been to prescribe a course of *Natrum-mur.* first, with the expectation that *Calc-carb.* would be needed later to complete the cure - in other words, to use a layers approach. This case though, presented an ideal opportunity to try out the group analysis method, so I studied the various permutations based on those basic components. *Calc-carb.* itself didn't quite fit the bill, and neither did *Natrum-mur.*or *Natrum-carb.* This left only one alternative, which was *Calc-mur.*, and I decided to give it as the first prescription. Interestingly, Scholten said that this particular remedy was especially indicated for people who found it hard to receive any care or nurturing from others, although they did in fact crave it. On questioning, this seemed to match the patient's internal state almost exactly. I gave her *Calc-mur.* 1M, and to my surprise she had a rapid and dramatic healing response on all levels, including a considerable weight loss without any change in dietary habits.

This first success spurred me on to try out many of the other combinations that Scholten described, and time after time I found his approach to yield good results. Not only was it helpful to have a range of new remedies to prescribe, but I found that my casetaking and case analysis were often enhanced by the information given in Sholten's book. By way of example, if a patient clearly had an issue with aggression - say it was someone who couldn't stand arguments or fights of any kind - then this would point immediately to the *Magnesium* group. With this in mind, I found it a fairly straightforward process to identify which of the *Magnesium* salts was required simply by questioning around that area of the person's life. If the issue was connected to the mother, then *Mag-mur.* would be the choice, if it was the father it would be *Mag-carb.*, and so on. I found this approach to be astonishingly simple once the basic

26

themes of each of the major components have been grasped.

I remember a case of someone who had a lot of resentment towards their partner, and for whom *Staphysagria* and *Natrum-mur.* had been given with only partial success. By combining the themes of resentment (*Ammonium* group) and partner (*Sulphuricum* group), the remedy *Ammonium-sulph.* was arrived at, which produced a fantastic result, despite my never having heard of it before!

I saw another case of a man who was afraid to enter into a relationship because his previous partner had left him, saying she thought he was childish and stupid (these were clearly things that he had come to believe were true). Combining the themes of childishness and stupidity (*Baryta* group) with partners (*Sulphuricum* group) I gave him *Baryta-sulph.* over a period of time, which helped his self-esteem in this area enormously.

I saw another case of a woman whose pre-occupation was to be seen by others as someone who was rich and successful. Combining the themes of worrying about what others think (*Calcium* group) with money and social status (*Fluoratum* group), the indicated remedy was *Calc-fluor.* Interestingly, she had a history of bony spurs and a tendency to dislocations, both of which are physical keynotes of the remedy. Needless to say she did very well on it. This, for me, was an example of how the group analysis method can enhance our knowledge of remedies that are already well-known in a certain area.

Once I had tried out many of the combinations introduced by Scholten, I found opportunity to prescribe other combinations which I hadn't even seen described. It was simply that a patient would present with a particular combination of features which suggested to me that a group analysis approach might prove useful. For example, I saw a man with a history of heart trouble and high blood pressure who had always been driven to succeed - all typical features of *Aurum*. In addition, however, he was extremely fastidious and had a high degree of anxiety about his health, bordering on hypochondria. This aspect suggested *Arsenicum* to me. Applying the group analysis method, I decided to give him *Aurum-arsenicosum* (without knowing anything about this particular remedy), which helped him a great deal in every area. Another man with an *Aurum*-type personality presented with asthma and low energy, plus he had a marked tendency to theorize and a number of physical keynotes suggesting *Sulphur*. On this rather unusual combination I prescribed *Aurum-sulph.*, again with a good result.

Recent Developments

Several years after the appearance of his first book, Sholten produced a follow-up volume entitled *Homeopathy and the Elements*. In this work, he took the idea of themes into the periodic table, identifying common threads and matching them to each of the series of elements to be found there. Again, the result has been an enormous number of new remedies and many new insights into familiar polychrests. Thus far my own experiments have been confined mostly to the mineral combinations outlined in Scholten's earlier book, and I recommend this first book as the best starting point for those who have no experience of using the group analysis method.

Further Reading

J.T. Kent
New Remedies & Lesser Writings
B. Jain Publishers, India

J. Scholten
Homeopathy and Minerals
Homeopathy and the Elements
Stitchting Alonissos, Utrecht, Netherlands

Intuitive Prescribing

It is time for the feminine, intuitve aspect in all of us to take its rightful place at the head of the table. The intuitive should be supported by the logical, not vice versa.

Arthur Bailey
Anyone can Dowse for Better Health

Definition
Prescribing from an immediate recognition or 'felt sense' of what is needed, without the intervention of the analytical mind.

Introduction
Intuition can take many forms and, whilst some homeopaths might object to my including it as a prescribing 'method', my reason for doing so is simply to acknowledge the fact that intuition has played a large part in my own casework and that of many of my colleagues over the years.

Skeptics and rationalists have often said to me that intuition works fine provided you have learnt all the relevant material beforehand. In other words, you will only have an intuition about a remedy you already know. My own experience has been that this is not entirely the case, and I am certainly open to the possibility that something completely new and previously unknown to me can pop into my awareness at any moment.

Intuition has a habit of arriving when you least expect it. Often it seems that it is necessary to go through a process of reasoning something out and analysing it in the usual way, but I have frequently found that when this process has failed to clarify things for me and I have given up in despair - that's the moment when intuition kicks in and offers a solution I would never have thought of, and sometimes a solution I have never even heard of!

Gut feelings and other phenomena
One thing that characterises intuition for me and differentiates it from other kinds of knowing, is that it is more of a general bodily experience. It seems a strange thing to claim that we can know something by way of a gut feeling or a feeling in the bones, but to me these are accurate descriptions of the way in which intuitive wisdom makes itself known.

The Yacqui Indian shamans of ancient Mexico recognised and identified several different ways of knowing, one of which they called 'direct knowledge'. They maintained that direct knowledge differs from everyday reasoning in as much as when it takes place, it creates the sensation of *knowing without knowing how you know*. This, to me, is what intuition is all about, and I firmly believe that we humans have the capacity to access knowledge directly without having the faintest idea where it came from.

That the whole body (not just the brain) is involved in intuitive knowing is demonstrated by techniques such as dowsing and applied kinesiology, which I will mention later. I can share an experience from my own practice, however, which alerted me to this fact some years ago.

I was struggling to find a remedy for a man complaining of back pain, with very few other symptoms to go on. One thing I sensed was that he carried a lot of unexpressed anger, and on this I decided to prescribe *Staphysagria* 10M. I wrote out the prescription and handed it to Beth, who was working for me in the clinic at this time, and whom I knew to be very intuitive. She made up the remedy, gave it to the patient and sent him on his way. Only then did she realise that she had given him not *Staphysagria* but *Stramonium* 10M. She said it was as if her hand had been pulled towards it, and she couldn't help herself.

I told her not to worry, as I hadn't been totally convinced that my prescription was accurate, and I figured that *Stramonium* had at least as much anger in its picture as *Staphysagria*. Needless to say, he had a return of vivid nightmares straight after taking it (which he hadn't told me about before), followed by a rapid improvement in his condition.

On another occasion, Beth brought a case to me that she needed help with. The moment I touched the folder holding the notes, I knew with absolute certainty *(without knowing how I knew it)* that the person in question needed *Mercurius*, which turned out to be the case.

Over the years I have witnessed and experienced many such intuitive knowings, and have come to believe that, like any other faculty, intuition is something that can certainly be developed with practice. The main requirement seems to be a willingness to listen to it, whatever form it takes, and to act on it. Some people get a voice in their head, others might see an image that reveals the indicated remedy. I know of homeopaths (and patients) who have had the remedy pop up and make itself known in their dreams.

Let the patient speak

Another aspect of intuitive prescribing that I want to mention is that when a practitioner and patient are attuned to each other, a field effect is created which seems to enhance the opportunities for intuition to manifest. This can take several forms. Once, for example, a patient to whom I had decided to give *Arsenicum* looked me right in the eye and asked, "what are you giving me then, *arsenic*?" Another patient declared that I would no doubt be giving her snake venom, which indeed was the case! I know of another patient who declared repeatedly during the interview that he was 'like granite'. No prizes for guessing what remedy he needed.

Children are especially good at intuiting their own remedies, and I have seen them do this successfully on countless occasions. This, for me, provides ample confirmation that we can know something intuitively that we have never consciously learned. I remember a colleague's young son self-prescribing *Vespa* for a badly inflamed sting, when *Apis* and other well-indicated remedies had failed. Another youngster, who was under three years old at the time, plucked *Eupatorium-perfoliatum* out of hundreds of remedy bottles and cured herself and some family members from a bad dose of 'flu.

On numerous occasions I have invited children to simply pick a remedy out of the box or off the shelf, and more often than not they are drawn immediately to the one they need. One child I remember pulled out *Syphilinum* 10M, which did more good than all the previous remedies that had been prescribed. Practitioners like me who have become accustomed to the idea that homeopathy by necessity involves hard labour find it difficult to accept that it really could be that simple, but children especially serve to remind us that the simplest solution is often the best one.

Dowsing

Many thousands of people have employed dowsing techniques to help diagnose health problems and to discover curative remedies. I worked in this way myself for a number of years, before my curiosity got the better of me and I wanted to know *why* a certain remedy worked for a certain patient. Interestingly, I found that as my materia medica knowledge grew, my ability to dowse accurately (or at least my *trust* in that ability) seemed to diminish accordingly.

Most dowsers use a pendulum to select remedies and it is simple enough once you have learned how to interpret your own responses. For me, a clockwise gyration meant 'yes', anti-clockwise meant 'no' and a back-and-forth swing meant 'can't answer' or 'rephrase the question', which usually turned out to be ambiguous in some way. Having ascertained what the different movements mean to you, and they do vary from person to person, the other requirement is to be able to phrase clear, unambiguous questions and to trust the responses that come. The pendulum has no real magical properties of its own, it is simply an extension of the practitioner's muscular and physiological system, and this system seems to 'know' when a remedy resonates with a person and when it doesn't.

In a letter to *The Homeopath*[1] Jay Yasgur writes of his experience dowsing for a remedy for a toe infection. His starting point was to ask whether the remedy he needed was in his kit - a pragmatic approach which I have used myself many times. The answer being yes, he then asked the pendulum to show which of the two columns of remedies in the list contained the one he needed. 'M-Z' came the reply. He then ran through that list alphabetically until the pendulum gave an unequivocal 'yes'. The remedy was *Sabadilla*, the only potency available was a 6x, which he took and it produced a beautiful cure.

As well as being able to suggest solutions that might not otherwise be considered, another advantage of dowsing is that it can be done just as effectively in the absence of the patient. Arthur Bailey, who has developed a wonderful set of flower essences[2] through dowsing, once prescribed a bottle of essences for me with no consultation whatsoever, working from a small hair sample which he used to 'tune in' to me whilst I was seventy miles away. The essences were so well chosen that I had an immediate healing response after the very first dose.

Many homeopaths use dowsing as a back-up tool to help differentiate between a group of possible remedies, or to help decide upon potency and repetition. The late Edward Whitmont talked of using a pendulum in this way. Dr. Grimmer, who was a colleague and contemporary of Kent, also employed dowsing techniques to discover remedies for his patients, as did another well-known American homeopath, Guy Beckley-Stearns.

Applied Kinesiology
If the pendulum is simply an extension of the muscular system, it stands to reason that there are other ways in which the body's responses to remedies and other substances can be determined. Stearns found through his research that the pupil would dilate markedly when a well-indicated remedy was brought into the energy field of a patient. In the 1960's, research pioneered in the U.S.A. by George Goodheart demonstrated that certain muscles will be instantaneously strengthened by an indicated remedy or other beneficial substance, and just as

immediately weakened by a toxin or substance to which the person is allergic. These discoveries opened up a whole new diagnostic field called applied kinesiology, or muscle-testing.

Kinesiology is simple to learn and, like dowsing, works very well as a confirmatory tool for homeopaths. Having decided upon a small group of possible remedies, it takes very little time to test them and see which one the body responds to most powerfully, and a similar process with a range of potencies will help determine the one that has the strongest resonance with the patient at that time.

Conclusion
It is in many ways an interesting time in the development of homeopathy. On the one hand, mainstream homeopathic education is becoming increasingly left-brain, academic and medically-aligned, and thousands of practitioners are dependent on computer programmes to assist them in their practice. On the other hand, there are a growing number of people developing the feminine, right-brain side of homeopathy, with the introduction of meditation and dream provings and a whole host of intuitive diagnostic and prescribing techniques. Hopefully these two branches will find ways to complement one another so that future homeopaths will learn both the art and science of homeopathy.

Further Reading
A. Bailey
Anyone can Dowse for Better Health
Quantum, W. Foulsham & Co. Ltd., Cippenham, Berks., England

M. La Tourelle &. A. Courtenay
Thorson's Introductory Guide to Kinesiology
Thorsons Publishers, England

C. Page
Beyond the Obvious - Bringing Intuition into our Awakening Consciousness
C.W. Daniel Co. Ltd., Saffron Walden, Essex, England

J. Thie
Touch for Health
Devorss Publications, California, U.S.A.

Isopathy

Definition

This term derives from the Greek *isos* meaning 'equal'. In homeopathic terminology, isopathy is usually taken to mean prescribing a remedy made from the supposed causative agents or products of a disease to a patient suffering that same disease. Thus for instance a patient with tuberculosis might be given *Bacillinum*, prepared from the sputum of another T.B. sufferer. If a remedy is made from the patient's own discharges or secretions which are then given back to that same patient (usually in potentised form), this is known as auto-isopathy. The method has also been expanded to include prescribing potencies of substances to which a patient is hypersensitive or allergic, such as wheat, milk, or a certain type of pollen.

Prescribing Technique

Various techniques have been described, ranging from a single dose of a high potency remedy to an injection of the patient's own blood in its crude state.

In a footnote to paragraph 56 of *The Organon*[1], Hahnemann asserts that the idea behind isopathy "contradicts all normal human understanding and hence all experience". He goes on to explain that if it has any validity at all then this is because the substance is altered by the potentisation process and therefore acts because it is *similar* rather than identical to the disease being treated. He may well be right in this respect, or it may be that isopathic remedies have their own unique sphere of action. Only further clinical work and close observation will make this clear.

Whilst some homeopaths would never resort to using isopathy, I have read numerous accounts of cases successfully treated by this method and have achieved some limited success with it myself, therefore I think it deserves a mention. Most practitioners (myself included) tend to keep it as a last resort for cases where all else has failed, or to use it as an adjunct to ordinary homeopathic treatment. Several authors have warned of the aggravations that can follow an auto-isopathic prescription, therefore these ought not to be used indiscriminately.

When to use Isopathy

Many patients are hypersensitive or allergic to certain substances or agents, and often these conditions are curable by traditional homeopathic methods. On occasion however, a patient will respond generally to homeopathic treatment but a specific allergy will remain uncured which may be problematic. In these cases isopathy can be a useful adjunct. Apart from this use, I could only otherwise recommend isopathy when all else has failed.

Case examples

I have treated patients with severe milk allergies which did not respond to constitutional and miasmatic treatment, but an occasional dose of *Lac vaccinum* or *Lac defloratum* produced a curative response. I have also given *Apis mellifica* in high potency to several people who were dangerously allergic to bee stings. One of these received no other homeopathic treatment, but found that when he was stung by bees subsequently he experienced only a normal local reaction, and being an apiarist this was of considerable benefit to him. I have also given potencies of the rape plant to hay fever sufferers who felt they were affected by the rape crops which are much in abundance, but so far have achieved only some palliative relief with this and no permanent cure. I recall reading a case of allergic reaction to strawberries where *Fragaria vesca* (potentised strawberry) was prescribed, following which the patient could eat them with impunity. Believe it or not, one of the symptomatic indications for *Fragaria* is a 'strawberry tongue'!

Dr. Eizayaga has stated that urinary tract infections such as cystitis are cured more quickly and permanently if the patient is given a potency prepared from their own urine together with the indicated remedy. He advises that if the 'infecting' organism present in the urine is isolated and cultured and that is then potentised, better results are obtained.

I once treated a man with severe, inveterate eczema which bled and wept terribly. On one occasion when we were both despairing of his recovery (and *Psorinum* didn't help!) he took a sample of his eruptions, had it potentised and took it. Whilst it didn't produce a cure, it seemed to afford him some relief and with further treatment his condition eventually cleared up.

I came across an interesting case of isopathy in an old edition of *The Homeopathic Recorder* (unfortunately I did not record the date). It told of a woman treated by Dr. Underhill Jr., whom he described as one of the worst cases of rheumatoid arthritis he had ever seen, and she also had a peculiar skin complaint. He tried numerous remedies without success, and eventually in desperation he had some potencies (30, 200, 1M) made from her blood and gave her those, again without success. The patient finally died uncured. Later the woman's daughter came to him for treatment for a skin complaint resembling ichthyosis. Dr. Underhill relates the story: "This (the skin condition) was so strikingly similar to that of her mother's condition, and she began to complain of pains in the joints, that the temptation to try her mother's potentised blood, on her, was too great for me and I gave it, and I got action. It flared her up terribly and laid her right up in bed, but I stuck to my guns and did nothing. I didn't dare repeat it and I didn't dare do anything else, and I let the case ride, so, after a terrific aggravation, she made a beautiful recovery and the ichthyosis has cleared up and never returned; but I have never dared give her another dose."

Whether the above response was due to symptom-similarity or because of the isopathic relationship is hugely debatable, but the result was certainly striking.

Impoderabilia
Some of our therapeutic agents classified as 'imponderable' have been used isopathically. *Electricitas* is said to have benefitted people who suffer tremendously from thunderstorms, and I know of a patient in whom it acted dramatically where indicated remedies failed, who had a history of having received numerous E.C.T. treatments. One wonders what it might do for those who are sensitive to overhead powerlines or who seem to attract excessive amounts of static electricity?

In a similar way, *Sol* has helped numerous patients who could tolerate little or no exposure to sunlight, and *Luna* is reported to have done the same for 'lunatics' and others affected adversely by the moon. I recently treated a patient who suffered with nightmares and disturbed sleep just before every full moon. I was toying with the idea of giving her *Luna*, but the rest of the picture suggested *Natrum mur.* which I gave and it cured the problem.

All of the above are examples of how isopathy may be helpful, mostly as an adjunct to other homeopathic methods. I have come across very little evidence that on its own isopathy will produce consistently curative results, but it will often tidy up the loose ends of a case in a way that nothing else can match.

There is a fairly broad consensus of opinion that disease nosodes do not on the whole act curatively when given for the disease to which they correspond. For instance, *Medorrhinum* is effective in suppressed gonorrhoea but not in acute gonorrhoea and *Carcinosin* seems better suited to pre-cancerous states that to patients with active cancer. Why this should be we can only speculate - perhaps homeopathy was never meant to be quite *that* simple?

Further Reading

I. Bernoville & G. Dano (Trans. from the French by R. Mukerji)
Nosodotherapy, Isopathy, Opotherapy
Pratap Homeo Pharmacy & Clinic, New Delhi, India

O. A. Julian
Treatise on Dynamised Micro-immunotherapy
Jain Publishing Co., New Delhi, India

Layers

Definition
A method based on the assumption that certain patients have distinct levels of dis-ease which require separate prescriptions to be given in appropriate sequence in order to bring about a complete and lasting cure.

Whilst several notable practitioners have acknowledged the existence of 'layered' cases, we are indebted to Dr. Eizayaga of Argentina for creating a coherent working model based around this idea.
See also: Sequential Prescribing

The Eizayaga Model
What follows is of course my own interpretation of Eizayaga's model based on my understanding of his teachings and my own experience in practice. Whilst some deviation from the original is inevitable, I hope that the spirit of Eizayaga's teaching has been maintained.

There are four main categories of layer to be considered:

1) Miasmatic layer
2) Constitutional layer
3) Fundamental layer
4) Lesion layer

Each of the above terms has a distinct meaning when used in the context of this model, and it is important not to confuse these meanings with other interpretations of the same words.

Below are the key components of each of the four major layers. The prescribing rules are different depending on which layer is being treated, so I have included these under each heading.

Constitutional Layer
This layer refers to what are basically *healthy* characteristics, and mostly they are genetic and immovable. These include the body type, hair colour, basic character/personality type, food desires and aversions, and general modalities such as relate to temperature and climate. All signs and symptoms on this level are compatible with good health & normality - they are neither pathological nor curable. The purpose of treatment on this layer is preventative, i.e. to strengthen

and fortify the constitution and thereby help to keep the person healthy. Only a few basic polychrest remedies are used, most notably *Sulphur, Calcarea carbonica, Silica, Phosphorus* and *Lycopodium*. As might be expected, babies and children are very commonly treated on this level, whereas most adults have acquired other layers which have to be removed before the underlying constitution can be treated.

How to Prescribe

Generally speaking, one or a few doses of the indicated remedy are given in a potency from the 30th upwards. The remedy may be repeated periodically in the same or a higher potency provided the person remains in good health.

Fundamental Layer

This layer refers mostly to *functional* symptoms on a mental, emotional or physical level. These are *acquired* characteristics, and can change throughout a person's life. Symptoms on this level relate to the person rather than to any disease process, but they are deviations from that person's healthiest state. This layer tends to overlap with the Kentian 'constitutional' picture, and the standard Kentian hierarchy of symptoms is usually applied (see *Constitutional Prescribing*). Commonly this layer is found to have resulted from an emotional ætiology such as grief, anger, fright etc. Food cravings and intolerances belong here, as these are not considered to be compatible with good health. All symptoms of this layer are generally reversible and curable. The purpose of the treatment is to remove functional disorders and to restore the patient to their original constitutional picture. Approximately thirty to forty polychrest remedies are most commonly used whose psychological pictures are well-defined, such as *Pulsatilla, Natrum mur., Stramonium, Aurum, Lachesis*, etc.

How to Prescribe

Eizayaga found from experience that many unnecessary aggravations were caused by giving the indicated remedy in too high a potency than was needed by the patient, and that the response obtained from the high potency was often unstable and liable to be antidoted. In order to overcome these disadvantages, he developed the following prescribing technique for use in treating the fundamental and lesional layers.

Cases should be commenced on a low potency (3c or 6c), given in repeated doses one to four times daily according to the severity of symptoms, sensitivity of the patient, level of drugging etc. The remedy is continued in this way for as long as the patient is seen to respond curatively to it. If an aggravation occurs (usually in the first few days), the frequency of dosage should be reduced accordingly, although minor aggravations will often disappear quickly without any adjustment of the potency or frequency.

When the remedy given ceases to elicit any further curative response, the case should be retaken to ascertain whether the same remedy is still indicated. If it is, then the same remedy is given in a higher potency and repeated daily as before, and this process is repeated as necessary. Thus for example, a patient might first be given *Pulsatilla* 6 tds; after 6 weeks it no longer helps so *Pulsatilla* 12 is given tds; if this ceases to act and the remedy is still indicated, *Pulsatilla* 18 or 30 is then given in repeated doses. In rare cases, a patient may be taken to the stage where they are receiving a remedy in the 200c or even higher, repeated on a daily basis. Provided the scale has been ascended gradually and systematically, no problems will result from this. In practice, it is far more common for a remedy to have achieved all that it can by the time the 30th potency has been reached.

If a remedy ceases to act and a new remedy picture is seen to emerge (other than the basic constitutional remedy), then the new remedy should be given in the same way as before, commencing at the lower end of the potency scale and gradually working up.

Lesion Layer
When a disease process has localised in a system, apparatus, organ or tissue, it is known as a lesion and may have to be treated separately from the other layers. A lesion may be either *acute* (e.g. appendicitis) or *chronic* (e.g. arthritis). It may be further categorised as *sporadic* (appearing at unpredictable intervals, e.g. gout); *periodic* (appearing at regular intervals or under predictable circumstances, e.g. asthma) or *permanent* (e.g. cancer). It may be reversible or irreversible, curable or incurable.

A lesion layer prescription is based upon the clinical diagnosis, the symptoms of the disease and all *local* modalities, concomitants and alternations. Thus the hierarchy of symptoms is the reverse of that used in constitutional prescribing. Only those mental & general symptoms are utilised which have appeared or become worse since the disease has existed. The purpose of the treatment is to remove the disease before curing the patient. Any remedy in the materia medica may be used, including organ remedies and those minor remedies having clinical indications only.

In some cases sub-lesions are added to the picture and may require treatment before the lesion layer itself can be tackled. For example, diabetes may be the lesion to be treated, but there are now added ulcers or visual impairment as a result of the diabetes. Similarly, a patient with cancer as the lesion layer may have just completed a course of chemotherapy or radiation, which can add a sub-lesion to the picture. The basic rule in lesional cases is always to start with the most recent and/or most limiting problem and to work back from there.

How to Prescribe
The guidelines for lesion layer prescribing are virtually identical to those that apply to the fundamental layer. As the vast majority of chronic lesional cases will have been subject to drugs and other treatments, the repeated-low-potency approach is extremely useful from the point of view of case management. I have found it is generally easier for the patient to withdraw allopathic drugs by this method without precipitating crises.

Miasmatic Layer
Five basic miasmatic or 'soil' types are recognised, each producing a predisposition to certain types of disease (a 'tendency to.............'). The general indications for each are given below:

Psora: skin problems, itch, seasonal allergies, problems with digestion, assimilation & elimination
Tuberculosis: respiratory problems, nasal, bronchial, pulmonary, allergies.
Sycosis: disorders of genitals, joints & mucous membranes, benign tumours, warts, catarrhal states, obsessions.
Syphilis: self-destructive tendencies, suicide, accidents, ulceration, necrosis, suppuration.
Cancer: morbidity, obsessiveness, suppressions, moles, pre-cancerous states.

The majority of people are deemed to have more than one miasm, and the rule of thumb is to treat the most active or uppermost first, as and when it is encountered. However, Eizayaga suggests that it is also a good policy to treat miasmatically *after* the patient is fully cured, in order to consolidate the cure and reduce the likelihood of a relapse.

There are three basic levels of activity that may apply to a miasm:

1) Dormant Miasm
This means that the miasm is indicated by the family history of the patient, or by the previous illnesses suffered by the patient, but there is no evidence that the miasm is active at the present time. The best approach with dormant miasms is to let sleeping dogs lie. If a dormant miasm is treated with the related

nosode it may be activated and, while this could be argued to be in the long-term interests of the patient, they are unlikely to see it that way.

2) Active Miasm

This means that the miasm is actively (i.e. currently) producing a tendency to certain problems, which continue to recur in spite of homeopathic treatment. An active miasm may also prevent well-indicated remedies from acting curatively or may provoke frequent and early relapses. This type of miasm should be treated with one or a few doses of the appropriate nosode in a potency from the 30th upwards. This is usually done intercurrently during treatment on another layer, and that treatment should be resumed, giving the same potency as had previously acted, shortly after the nosode has been given. The purpose of the intercurrent miasmatic treatment is to reduce the activity of the miasm so that indicated remedies may be given with greater benefit.

3) Exposed Miasm

When a miasm is exposed, this means that the picture presenting is of the corresponding nosode - that is to say, the patient is presenting a clear picture of, say *Medorrhinum* or *Tuberculinum*, with the mental state, food desires and other characteristic symptoms of the remedy. This is the only time in this model when a major nosode would be given as a *first* remedy, and Eizayaga recommends it be given in these cases using the ascending potency scale described above. Thus you might prescribe *Tub. bov.* 6 tds, increasing to *Tub. bov.* 12 as required, and so on.

Other Layers

If a patient has 'never been well since' a specific disease, the acquired miasmatic layer should be treated with the corresponding disease nosode in the same way as an active miasm would be treated. Usually a few doses of the remedy in a medium or high potency are all that is required. The same procedure should be followed to deal with a drugs layer where this is obscuring the layers underneath.

Drawbacks

The main drawback with this method is that it can sometimes be difficult to ascertain when a lesional prescription is required in favour of a fundamental layer prescription. In many cases this is fairly obvious, such as in active cancer or acute asthma - here the disease quite clearly has a 'life of its own' and there are usually clearcut symptoms and modalities of the disease on which to prescribe. The difficulty is more often encountered with diseases such as eczema, psoriasis and arthritis, where the symptoms of both patient and disease can be closely interwoven.

I have found from experience that wherever there is any doubt as to whether there is a separate lesional layer in a case, it is a good policy to try and find a remedy that covers both patient *and* disease first of all. It is also extremely helpful to go over the symptoms of the case carefully and ask the patient how long each of them has been present. If a number of symptoms appeared at around the same time in a person's life, often that indicates that a layer was acquired at that point, especially if a grief or other trauma had occurred a short time before.

When to Use the Method
The layers approach is most appropriate in cases with advanced pathologies, particularly the degenerative diseases, and in cases complicated with drugs. It is also well suited to complex cases showing multiple ætiologies and a profusion of indicated remedies. It is sometimes surprising how complex and confusing cases may be untangled and made sense of by separating out the layers. I would also consider using this approach in any case expressing symptoms of the disease rather than of the patient.

It is generally inappropriate to use this method in cases showing a clearly-defined single remedy image. In the Eizayaga model, such cases can be interpreted as having several layers, each of which requires the same remedy. This seems to me an unnecessary complication of cases which, by their nature, are uncomplicated and easy to treat by the constitutional approach.

Case Examples

Case One
This first example shows the breakdown of a complex, chronic case which is ideal for the layers method. Cases like this illustrate the futility of attempting to find a single remedy that will take care of everything, as is recommended by some constitutional prescribers. Overleaf is an abbreviated chronological 'timeline' I constructed for the patient who was suffering from the effects of heart failure when I first saw him:

What this patient presented with was "never been well since influenza", but as is often the case this was only the tip of a very large iceberg. Nonetheless, an ætiological prescription of *Influenzinum* set him on the road to recovery. This was followed by several months treatment with *Crataegus* Ø which restored his heart to normal function. After this his gout returned to its original site and required prolonged treatment with *Urtica urens* Ø before it finally subsided. Only at this stage in the treatment did he present a clear fundamental layer picture - initially *Nux vomica* and later *Arsenicum album*, following which he received prolonged constitutional and miasmatic treatmen

This case shows clearly the progression inwards of disease following allopathic suppression, which is often a major ætiological factor in chronic cases.

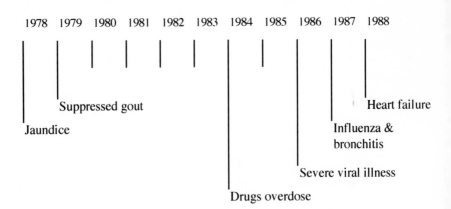

Case Two
This second case illustrates how an active miasm will superimpose symptoms of the miasm onto other layers of the case, creating confusion for the prescriber attempting to find a single remedy.

A nineteen year old woman, presenting with severe hay fever, constantly for several weeks; which has recurred every year since the age of thirteen. This is how I saw the structure of the case at the first visit:

Lesion layer   Fluent coryza
                                Bland lachrymation
                                Itching eyes - must rub
                                Wheezing < evening & night
                                > sitting up, > fresh air

Indicated remedy: *Pulsatilla*

Fundamental layer	Low thirst
	Low energy < on waking
	Weeps easily;
	> for weeping
	Averse fats & pork
	Dysmenorrhoea
Indicated remedy:	*Pulsatilla*
Constitutional layer	Tall, slender build, Chilliness
	Empty & weak from hunger
	Fears something will happen
	Extroverted and open personality
	Desires salt
Indicated remedy:	*Phosphorus*
Miasmatic layer	Recurrent hay fever
	Allergies to wheat & milk
	Reacts badly to insect bites
	Neck glands frequently swollen
	Family history: hay fever; allergies;
	eczema; asthma
Indicated remedy:	*Tuberculinum (& Psorinum)*

Pulsatilla 6 t.d.s. was prescribed, which resulted in a severe aggravation of the symptoms on the second day, together with total malaise and a feeling that she had influenza. She continued taking the remedy, and on the third day all the hay fever symptoms disappeared and the flu-like feeling had gone. Following this, her general energy improved and her periods became less painful. When there was no further response to *Pulsatilla* (after about 7 weeks), the case was retaken and *Tuberculinum* seemed better indicated than *Phosphorus* on the remaining symptoms. *Tuberculinum bovinum* was given in high potency at long intervals, with marked improvement in the allergic and the hypoglycæmic symptoms. She then discontinued treatment. The hay fever returned the following year but a lot milder than before, and it responded instantly to a few doses of *Pulsatilla* 12.

This case illustrates how the layers do not always present in a pre-determined sequence, and the practitioner should be prepared to prescribe on whatever picture emerges following the removal of each layer.

Prescribing out of Sequence

Sometimes I have prescribed a remedy in the Kentian manner based on the emotional and general symptoms and de-emphasising the symptoms of the disease. Occasionally the result has been that a prolonged and severe aggravation of the disease symptoms occurs without any subsequent amelioration. Sometimes the patient will report improvement in some general area, but the disease state has clearly progressed. In the Kentian model, this response tends to be interpreted as an incurable case, and an antidotal or palliative remedy is sought. I find it more fruitful to interpret this response as being indicative of a *layered* case, which requires that the disease (lesion layer) be treated first before treating the patient (fundamental and constitutional layers). Such a response is helpful in the sense it indicates that the remedy given was definitely indicated on a deep level - it was simply given out of sequence.

Prescribing for any layer at an inappropriate time will tend to produce an inappropriate response - that is, something may happen but it wasn't quite what you had in mind. The following case illustrates this.

Case Three

A woman complained of a Bartholin (vaginal) cyst causing some pain and discomfort. She was worried it might turn cancerous and had a fear of cancer generally. She had a tendency to frequent colds and hay fever recurrently every year. Hard working; had always been overweight. Her breasts became swollen and tender before each period; periods tended to be early. Recurrent patches of eczema in the bends of her joints.

This patient appeared to require the same remedy for both the fundamental and constitutional layers, and the local problem had not developed to a stage where it could be considered a lesion. A single dose of *Calcarea carbonica* 200 was prescribed and was followed by a reduction in the size and discomfort of the cyst, she felt more relaxed generally and her periods were improved. Then she developed flu-like symptoms for several days and after this a dry cough at night.

As the cough seemed to be persisting and her miasmatic background was predominantly tubercular, she was given *Tuberculinum* in ascending collective single dose (30-200-1M). The result was that within a few days she was thrown into a state of emotional turmoil. She was weeping uncontrollably, thought she was losing her mind and felt totally grief-stricken, although she didn't know why. She started having panic attacks where she would feel faint, shaky and couldn't get her breath. She had severe pins and needles in her hands. She was terrified to take any further remedies in case she became even worse.

Abundant reassurance was given and *Ignatia* 6 was sent to be taken three times daily as needed. Within a few days calm was restored and she continued to improve generally without further medicine. *Tuberculinum* had obviously been indicated on a miasmatic level to produce such a dramatic response, but the likelihood is that it was given prematurely.

Cases like that above serve to remind one how benevelont homeopathy really is. Even when you apparently 'get it wrong', the organism invariably responds by showing you exactly what needs to be done and presents you with a golden opportunity to sort things out. Layers can sometimes be well-camouflaged and it is advisable to always be prepared to adjust or even abandon your initial perception of a case as the treatment progresses.

Further Reading

I. Watson
Therapeutics & Layers
Recorded Seminar, available in Audiotape and CD formats
www.ianwatsonseminars.com

Miasmatic Prescribing

All chronic diseases of mankind, even those left to themselves, not aggravated by a perverted treatment, show, as said, such a constancy and perseverance, that as soon as they have developed and have not been thoroughly healed by the medical art, they evermore increase with the years, and during the whole of man's lifetime; and they cannot be diminished by the strength belonging even to the most robust constitution. Still less can they be overcome and extinguished. Thus they never pass away of themselves, but increase and are aggravated even till death. They must therefore all have for their origin and foundation constant chronic miasms, whereby their parasitical existence in the human organism is enabled to continually rise and grow.

Samuel Hahnemann
Chronic Diseases

Definition

Miasma = defilement, pollution
This method is based on the assumption that there exists in virtually everyone an inherited or acquired energy blockage or disturbance producing a predisposition towards a particular and recognizable pattern of illness. Implicit in this method is the idea formulated by Hahnemann that it is impossible to fundamentally and permanently cure a chronic disease state unless treatment is directed towards the underlying miasm(s).

Prescribing Technique

There are two main variants of this method. The first involves the use of nosodes (remedies from the products of disease or diseased tissues) whilst the second employs 'traditional' remedies which are known to have a particular relationship to the miasm in question. The actual prescribing techniques are variable according to which of these approaches is taken.

The use of Nosodes

Some homeopaths consider that nosodes are no different to any other remedies and that there are no grounds for prescribing them other than symptom-similarity. I feel that this is a somewhat narrow viewpoint which denies the bulk of clinical experience. There is abundant evidence that nosodes have certain specific areas of use and that they may be indicated in a variety of different ways. It should also be noted that the nosodes are inadequately represented in the repertories, so that if repertorisation is taken as the basis for the prescription then a nosode is most unlikely to be prescribed. This is in contradiction to my own and other homeopaths' experience that the nosodes are in fact amongst the most frequently indicated remedies.

The five major miasmatic nosodes are *Psorinum, Medorrhinum, Syphilinum, Tuberculinum* and *Carcinosin*. Below are given the different situations in which a major nosode ought to be considered.

Nosode is indicated remedy: Nosodes such as *Psorinum* or *Tuberculinum* are often indicated and prescribed as remedies in their own right, based on the presenting symptom picture. Bearing in mind that they do not feature prominently in the repertories, it is an absolute necessity for the prescriber to become thoroughly acquainted with the nosode remedy pictures.

Indicated remedies fail: When well-selected remedies fail to act, this may indicate the presence of an active miasm which requires treatment with the appropriate nosode. It should of course be remembered that 'well-selected' is a relative term, and the prescription of a nosode is only one of the options that should be considered in the event of a non-response. A 'lack of reaction' has traditionally been considered to be evidence of a psoric taint, but in fact any of the miasms seem to be capable of inhibiting the action of indicated remedies.

Patient relapses: Sometimes the remedy given produces a response in the patient but it is short-lived and is followed by a quick return to the patient's former state. Another possibility is that the symptom picture becomes altered after each prescription but the basic disease tendency is left uncured. Either event may require a nosode in order to to bring about fundamental and lasting improvement.

Acute disease fails to resolve: If an acute disease lingers on and the patient appears to lack the vitality to throw it off completely, even with the help of indicated remedies, often a nosode will provide the necessary stimulus and clear the condition up. Clarke observed that influenza often seemed to waken up the tubercular miasm, and he found that *Tuberculinum Koch* was the best remedy to clear up lingering cases[1]. Foubister discovered that both whooping cough and glandular fever could often be cleared up by a few doses of *Carcinosin* when they failed to resolve[2].

Miasm obscures symptom-picture: Some cases present such an overwhelming miasmatic tendency that it stands out as the dominant feature of the case. In these cases it will sometimes pay dividends to prescribe a nosode as a first remedy, with the expectation that a clearer remedy-image will arise and a good response will be obtained when that remedy has been given. Having prescribed symptomatically-indicated remedies in these type of cases and seen several remedies 'bounce off' the patient, I find this strategy a useful time-saver.

I treated a six year-old boy diagnosed as having porphyria, the chief elements of the case being that he had pink urine, pink teeth, and a severe intolerance to light, particularly sunlight, such that his skin just fell off him after a short exposure. The main thing that struck me about him was his physical appearance - he had a large, neanderthal-style head and could be best described as goblin-like. After several unsuccessful attempts at finding a symptomatically-similar remedy, I decided to forget the symptoms and deal with the hefty miasmatic load he was carrying. The nature of his disorder and his general appearance suggested *Syphilinum* (although the family history was predominantly tubercular), which produced a definite improvement in his skin condition, but the underlying disease state remained uncured.

Interestingly, the remedy-picture that emerged afterwards was *Tuberculinum*, to which he also responded. Homeopaths long ago made the observation that as one miasm becomes subdued, another will often be seen to come to life and the miasmatic basis of the treatment will have to be changed accordingly. This is confirmed by the fact that all of the major nosodes are closely related to one another and in many instances are complementary, one taking up the work where another has left off.

The Use of Anti-Miasmatic Remedies

All of the deeper acting remedies have been credited with anti-miasmatic properties, ever since Hahnemann recognised the relationship between psora and *Sulphur*. It is therefore considered possible to treat on a miasmatic level by employing remedies that are similar to the miasm, as well as or even instead of to the symptoms. In Kent's *Repertory* there are rubrics representing the syphilitic and sycotic miasms - strangely, psora has been excluded, but this rubric can be found in the *Synthetic Repertory* of Barthel and Klunker. The best way to use these rubrics seems to be to take the dominant miasmatic tendency of the patient as the equivalent of one characteristic symptom, and to include the corresponding rubric in the repertorisation.

Hahnemann's method

At the time that Hahnemann was practising in Paris with his new wife Melanie (1835-43), his observation was that psora was the predominant miasm. Such was its prevalence, he felt it necessary to treat virtually every chronic case with *Sulphur*, this being the major anti-psoric remedy. His preferred method[3] , worked out after years of experimentation, was to give *Sulphur* usually at the outset, either as an LM potency or a centesimal potency (up to 200) diluted in water and alcohol and repeated at regular intervals such as daily or every other day. He would continue with this until such time as new symptoms came up or certain symptoms intensified, when he would then prescribe for the new symptoms immediately with the best indicated remedy. He would either stop the *Sulphur* while doing so, or in some cases would continue to give it, say in an LM potency continuously, while treating the new aspect of the disorder with a different remedy in a centesimal potency. The evidence suggests that Hahnemann prescribed *Sulphur* in this way even in cases where it did not seem at all indicated by the symptoms, so it is clear he was prescribing on miasm-similarity rather than symptom-similarity.

Determining the Dominant Miasm

I take as my overall starting point that as far as inherited predispositions go, most of us have a fair sized pinch of just about everything, so it is more often a case of "how much" rather than "which?" Just as multiple remedy images are often seen to overlap in the same patient, miasms are seen to do likewise and the art is in determining where the emphasis lies at the time of treatment. There are several factors to be taken into account in determining the dominant miasm.

Family history: When there is a prevalence of certain diseases in the ancestors of the patient, this can give clues as to the probable miasmatic inheritance.

Personal medical history: The pattern of illnesses throughout a patient's life, including the presenting disorder, can usually be matched to a particular miasmatic disposition.

Remedies which have acted well: If the remedies to which the patient has previously reacted are all of a similar miasmatic tendency, that miasm is probably predominant. Supposing *Thuja, Staphysagria* and *Natrum sulph.* have all produced a good response, the sycotic miasm is probably predominant and *Medorrhinum* is likely to be the best indicated nosode.

Acquired Miasms

So far we have concentrated on inherited disease tendencies, which in practice are those most commonly encountered. It also occurs, however, that a miasm may be acquired during a person's lifetime in one of several ways. Firstly, following an attack of acute disease, if a chronic disease tendency emerges then an acquired miasm is a possibility. If, for example, a person has never regained their health following an attack of chicken pox, that may be an acquired miasm and will often respond to a dose of the appropriate nosode, which in this case would be *Varicella*. All of the acute disease nosodes such as *Morbillinum, Parotidinum, Influenzinum* etc. may be used in this way. Dr. M. L. Tyler made widespread use of these acute disease nosodes in her practice and some remarkable case examples are to be found in her writings.

There is also evidence to suggest that miasms may be 'contracted' by one individual from another, assuming of course that a susceptibility already exists in the individual affected. I have seen this occur most clearly in relation to the sycotic miasm, which appears to be transferable by sexual contact. This does not mean that the person becomes infected with gonorrhoea, which laboratory tests will generally confirm has not taken place.

Case Example
A woman aged thirty-one presented with a persistent vaginal discharge, which was profuse, brown, sometimes bloody, and very offensive "as if something had gone off". It seemed to start about two years previously with a 'vaginal infection' which was treated with antibiotics. The soreness had cleared up but the discharge became offensive and continuous. Apart from this her general health had been and remained excellent - she ate a macrobiotic diet, practised yoga regularly and looked a picture of health. The only other symptom of note was a flat wart on the back of her left hand, which had been there for years.

Her general and emotional symptoms suggested *Lycopodium*, but it didn't seem sufficiently well indicated, nor did it cover the symptoms of her chief complaint particularly well. Instead, I took the particulars of the discharge and prescribed *Kreosotum* 30, with the result that the discharge cleared up dramatically but just as quickly returned when she stopped the remedy - in other words it palliated rather than cured.

On her return visit I decided to question further for an aetiology, and discovered that the discharge had appeared a few months after she had started a new relationship. As far as she was aware, her new partner had no history of gonorrhoea, but she couldn't be sure. Either way, it seemed like a case of acquired sycosis and on this basis I prescribed *Medorrhinum* 200. Her period came on early soon after the remedy and was unusually heavy, but as the period subsided so did the discharge and it never returned.

Whether a miasm can truly be acquired, or whether it is simply awoken from a dormant state is open to debate. In the above case there was nothing in the family history and virtually nothing in the patient's personal history to suggest latent sycosis. I have subsequently treated a number of patients who have 'never been well since' a change of partner or since getting married, and *Medorrhinum* has been the curative remedy for several of them. One such was a woman in her seventies of previous good health, who had remarried at the age of sixty-eight and developed appalling rheumatoid arthritis shortly afterwards. After *Medorrhinum* she discharged green pus from her nose and throat for several weeks whilst her joints improved dramatically.

New Miasms?

Homeopaths have speculated that the three miasms discovered by Hahnemann (psora, sycosis & syphilis) have become engrafted upon one another to such an extent that the 'new' miasms of tuberculosis and cancer are the result. Clinical experience certainly supports the view that these new miasms exist, and *Tuberculinum* and *Carcinosin* are now indispensable additions to the materia medica. It seems unlikely that the story has ended there, and we should be open to the possibility that there will be other miasms to contend with in the future. One author[4] has stated that radiation, heavy metal and petro-chemical miasms are already producing a myriad of pathological tendencies, and to me this seems perfectly credible.

Activity of Miasms

Viewed on a wide scale, miasms appear to have cycles of activity, much like epidemics of acute disease, with a prodromal period, a peak and then a decline. Hahnemann noted psora as being predominant, with sycosis and syphilis far less prevalent. European and American homeopaths practising in the late 1800's and early 1900's observed that the tubercular miasm started to predominate. Following this, the sycotic miasm enjoyed a period of great activity. In the present day, there is evidence that the cancer miasm is heading towards a peak of activity, certainly in the so-called 'developed' nations, whilst the sycotic and tubercular miasms are still very much in evidence. The syphilitic miasm has been relatively overshadowed throughout this period, yet by no means has it expired completely - indeed there is evidence emerging which suggests a strong link between A.I.D.S. and suppressed syphylis[5]. That A.I.D.S. may be closely linked to the syphilitic miasm seems probable as the remedies most commonly indicated in A.I.D.S. patients have been the anti-syphilitics such as *Arsenicum album*, *Mercurius* and *Nitric acid*.

Genetic Diseases

If we accept Hahnemann's theory of inherited miasms as being plausible, then all of the disorders considered to be 'genetic' by orthodox medicine must be treated as having a miasmatic basis. Certainly it seems true that children born, for example, with Down's syndrome or cystic fibrosis will invariably have indications for one and usually several nosodes during the course of treatment.

Levels of Activity

Dr. Eizayaga has clarified the different levels of activity that a miasm may manifest. These are related under the chapter on 'Layers Method'.

Further Reading

J. H. Allen
The Chronic Miasms Psora and Pseudo-Psora (2 Vols.)
Jain Publishing Co., New Delhi, India

H. C. Allen
Materia Medica of the Nosodes
Jain Publishing Co., New Delhi, India

D. M Foubister
The Carcinosin Drug Picture
Indian Books & Periodicals Syndicate, New Delhi, India

S. Hahnemann
The Chronic Disease: Their Peculiar Nature and Their Homeopathic Cure
Jain Publishing Co., New Delhi, India

R. D. Micklem
Carcinosin: A Compendium of References
R. D. Micklem, Queensbury, Bradford

P. S. Ortega
Notes on the Miasms
National Homeopathic Pharmacy, New Delhi, India

H. A. Roberts
The Principles and Art of Cure by Homeopathy
Jain Publishing Co., New Delhi, India

P. Speight
A Comparison of the Chronic Miasms
Health Science Press, Saffron Walden, Essex

I Watson
Understanding the Miasms
Recorded Seminar, available in Audiotape and CD formats
www.ianwatsonseminars.com

Organ Remedies

And we thus see that organ-remedies by restoring the disturbed organ to health, cure the organism itself

James Compton-Burnett

Synonyms: Organ Supports; Drainage; Organopathy

Definition
This method is based on the assumption that a) certain remedies have a specific affinity for certain organs, and b) there are patients in whom it is desirable or necessary to treat specific organs or systems in order that the whole person may be properly cured.

History & Development
Paracelsus (1490-1541) made great practical use of the idea that each organ of the body has its counterpart in nature. In traditional herbal medicine many substances have found their way into use by the application of the *Doctrine of Signatures*, whereby the plant's shape, colouring, habitat and other features have been utilised as guides to its therapeutic applications. The common names of many medicinal plants betray their organ-affinities quite clearly - Eyebright (*Euphrasia*), Liver-wort (*Hepatica*), Knitbone (*Symphytum*), Lung-wort (*Sticta*), Chaste-tree (*Agnus castus*), Squaw-root (*Caulophyllum*) and Blood-root (*Sanguinaria*). In virtually every case, these original observations have been confirmed when the remedies have been proved and introduced into homeopathic practice.

Rademacher
Practising in Germany in the early Nineteenth century, Rademacher developed his own therapeutic system, independent of the radical new system being introduced by Hahnemann and his followers. He was largely an empiricist using both traditional and original remedies, and throughout his writings he acknowledges his debt to Paracelsus, from whom he drew much of his inspiration.

Rademacher was able to distinguish clearly between "universal remedies" which were needed to treat the whole person, and "organ remedies" which were needed to treat individual parts. His experience taught him that many diseases were entirely dependent upon the imbalance within a specific organ, and as such could be entirely cured by a remedy that would restore the proper function of that organ. He stressed that organ remedies would only cure *primary* affections of the organ in question, and accurate assessment of the source of organ diseases was essential. Thus, for example, if respiratory symptoms were secondary to a disorder of the liver, it was a liver remedy that was required. He advised that in cases where the origin of an organ disease was doubtful, particularly where abdominal pain was a feature, attention should be paid to the region where the very last remnant of pain lingers at the end of an attack. Here, he says, will the organ that is primarily affected be found.

Rademacher stated that universal remedies would only cure true affections of the whole organism, and not sympathetic ones originating from a diseased organ. Similarly, organ remedies would only cure genuine organ diseases, and not diseases of the whole person which happened to manifest primarily in certain organs.

It is worth noting that according to the translator of Rademacher's writings, A. A. Ramseyer, the original German writings of Rademacher extended to two large volumes of over 800 pages each, and ran to four editions. The English version, whilst enlightening, consists of just 100 pages, which obviously leaves a great deal of treasure still lying buried. Hopefully this potential mine of information will be fully explored in the near future.

Burnett
James Compton Burnett took up the work of organ prescribing in England in the late nineteenth century and placed it in a homeopathic context. He pointed out the difference between prescribing on the basis of symptom-similarity and on the basis of organ-similarity, both of which he regarded as equally valid applications of the law of similars, each to be used as appropriate to the case. We are fortunate to have Burnett's writings available in print, giving many detailed accounts of the use of organ remedies in his own cases.

Burnett freely admits to taking most of his inspiration from the work of Paracelsus and Rademacher, but he was able to clarify the indications for many of the remedies he found recommended for use in treating certain organs. Examples would be *Carduus marianus*, *Chelidonium* and *Ceanothus*. Burnett was amply qualified to develop this work because, apart from being a highly skilled homeopath he was also a master diagnostician, able by palpation and observation to accurately assess the areas of organ weakness in each individual.

French Contributions

On the continent, the French homeopaths Nebel, Vannier, Julian and others have contributed much to the field of organ therapeutics in homeopathy. They introduced the concept of 'drainage' whereby organs or systems are detoxified and toned up before administering the indicated constitutional remedy, primarily to avoid unnecessary aggravations. They have also done a great deal of work on the use of sarcodes and sarcode-derivatives, particularly those derived from the endocrine glands.

Prescribing Technique

Usually low potencies (up to 6x) or mother tinctures are employed in organ prescribing, and the degree of symptom-similarity may be negligible. I generally follow Burnett's guidance and prescribe mother tinctures at the rate of five drops in a little water to be taken three times daily. Two drops per dose is usually sufficient for children. Occasionally I have used fluid extracts obtained from a reliable herbal suppliers in place of homeopathically prepared mother tinctures, and find that they serve the purpose equally well. If these are prescribed, usually two or three drops for each dose will prove sufficient owing to their high concentration.

If a patient who is taking a mother tincture experiences any new symptoms, this is usually a sign that the remedy is well indicated but the dosage is too high. A reduction in the amount prescribed will generally produce the required curative response without any discomfort. I have had several patients state that they felt slightly queasy soon after taking *Cratægus* Ø for heart trouble, and they all responded well to the remedy without further problems when the number of drops was reduced from five to two per dose. My suspicion is that when a patient is sensitive to a tincture in this way it is probably indicated on symptom-similarity as well as having the organ affinity.

My personal preference is always to prescribe an organ remedy on its own before commencing treatment on other levels. In doing this there can be no question as to the effects of the organ remedy, and I have often been surprised by the results. Some practitioners prefer to give the indicated constitutional remedy in high potency and the organ remedy in tincture or low potency simultaneously and, while I have no quibbles with this technique, I find that opportunities for learning are often lost by doing so. In some cases urgency will demand that several aspects must be tackled at once, but for me this is an exception rather than the rule.

Sarcodes

Organ prescribing incorporates the use of sarcodes & sarcode-derivatives (potentised healthy organs & their secretions) e.g. *Thyroidinum, Insulin, Adrenalin* etc. There is abundant clinical evidence that organs can be acted upon therapeutically by potencies either of the organ itself or of its secretions. Some of these sarcodes have been prepared from the corresponding organ in an animal - *Thyroidinum* for instance was taken from the dried thyroid gland of the sheep. Others have been prepared from human tissues taken from laboratory specimens.

According to French research, different potencies of the same substance have different uses therapeutically. Thus *Folliculinum*, for instance, is said to *arouse* organ function in 3x or 4c potencies, whilst in the 7c it will *regulate* function and in the 9c it will *inhibit*.

Uses of Sarcodes

I generally tend to use herbal organ support remedies in preference to sarcodes for mostly aesthetic reasons, but there are certain situations when a sarcode is indispensable. Firstly, they are useful when patients have had an organ or part of an organ damaged, destroyed or surgically removed. As an example, I treated a boy who had a brain tumour removed and who recovered generally but his growth was stunted. This was thought due to the tumour having impinged upon his pituitary gland. Constitutional treatment helped him generally but didn't affect his growth, which was the main problem. Consequently I gave him *Pituitrin* 30, once weekly at first and then less frequently over a period of many months, and he started to grow normally soon after starting the remedy.

Sometimes a sarcode will be useful when an organ has been subdued by the use of drugs, a good example being the adrenal glands following treatment with corticosteroids. The resulting energy depletion can be devastating following the withdrawal of steroids, but the recovery may be hastened by prescribing *Adrenal whole gland* in low potency over a period of weeks or a few months.

Patients who are dependent on a drug to replace the secretion of a diseased organ can sometimes be enabled to reduce the dosage to a minimum or completely withdraw the drug by substituting an appropriate sarcode. For example, I have seen myxoedemic patients who were able to reduce or withdraw thyroxine by substituting *Thyroidinum* in a low potency. Sometimes with further treatment the sarcode can be later withdrawn, but in other cases where the organ function cannot be restored it must be continued at a maintenance dosage. Dr. Muzumdar of India has obtained encouraging results[1] with diabetic patients using potencies of *Insulin*. I am sure there is a vast field of research here which ought to be more widely explored. Many patients who are considered incurable by other means, including more traditional homeopathic methods, might well have a different prognosis if we knew how to utilise sarcodes and other organ remedies more effectively.

Some Leading Organ Remedies
Below are some of the leading organ remedies which I use regularly in practice. Where more than one is listed, the symptoms of the case should be used to determine the choice. The remedies listed in bold type are those which I find most useful in cases of straightforward organ weakness or dysfunction, where there are no distinguishing symptoms calling for a particular organ remedy.

This list of remedies (and potencies) is intended to be suggestive rather than definitive, my general policy being to omit anything which I haven't used, or seen used, in practice. I am aware that we all have our favourites, however, and would welcome contibutions from readers who have found other organ remedies to be equally or more useful than the ones I have listed. I have generally omitted to include major polychrest remedies, trusting that the reader will be familiar with their respective organ affinities.

Brain & Nervous System	**Avena sativa Ø,** Kali phos. 6x Hypericum 6-CM
Heart	**Cratægus Ø,** Strophanthus Ø, Cactus Ø, Adonis vernalis Ø, Convallaria Ø
valves	Spongia 6, Naja 6
Digestive organs	Alfalfa Ø, Hydrastis Ø
stomach	**Hydrastis Ø**
Liver & gall-bladder	**Chelidonium Ø-3x,** Carduus marianus Ø, Taraxacum Ø, Cholesterinum 6x-200, Hydrastis Ø-6x, Mag. mur. 6
Spleen	**Ceanothus Ø-6,** Quercus Ø
Urinary organs	Berberis vulg. Ø, Uva-ursi Ø
kidneys	**Berberis vulg. Ø,** Solidago 3x
bladder	**Equisetum Ø,** Triticum rep. Ø

Female organs	
breast	Phytolacca Ø-CM
uterus	Fraxinus Am. Ø, Helonias Ø-6, Caulophyllum 6x-10M Thlaspi bursa pastoris Ø
ovaries	Folliculinum 6-30, Oophorinum 30

Male organs	**Agnus castus Ø,** Selenium 6 Caladium 6
prostate	**Sabal serrulata3x,** Thuja 6x, Conium 6, Pulsatilla 6x, Ferrum picricum 6

Blood (general toxicity)	**Echinacea Ø,** Gunpowder 6x, Pyrogen 6-200, Baptisia 3x-200

Veins	**Hamamelis Ø-30,** Vipera 12, Pulsatilla 6x, Calc-fluor 12x

Arteries	Baryta mur 6x, Cratægus Ø

Skin (general underfunction)	**Berberis aquifolium Ø,** Lappa arctium Ø, Skookum chuck 3x-12x

Bones	**Symphytum Ø,** Calc. phos. 6x Heckla lava 6, Phosphorus 6

Endocrine glands	
pituitary	Pituitrin 6-30, Baryta carb. 30
thyroid	**Fucus vesic. 3x,** Iodum 6-30, Thyroidinum 6
adrenals	Adrenal gland 6, Adrenalin 6
pancreas	Phosphorus 6, Iris vers. 6x

Multiple Affinities

Some organ remedies have more than one specific affinity and these combined affinities can be made use of where a similar combination presents in a patient. Here are some examples:

Respiratory & Gastric organs	Lobelia-inflata Ø, Grindelia 3x
Respiratory & Heart	Spongia 6, Iodum 6
Uterus & Urinary organs	Thlaspi-bursa-past. Ø
Kidneys & Liver	Berberis-vulgaris Ø
Heart & Liver	Digitalis 6-30, Aurum met. 6
Heart & Kidneys	Spartium Ø, Strophanthus Ø, Eel-serum 6

When to use Organ Remedies

My own experience suggests to me that organ support remedies ought to be much more widely used than at present, as the method carries many advantages. Firstly, there are patients whose entire symptomatology revolves around weakness or dysfunction of a particular organ. In these cases the organ weakness may present an obstacle to the cure and often it will be found that indicated constitutional remedies do not perform as well as they ought until the weakness is rectified. These are what Rademacher would consider primary organ diseases, and sometimes when an organ remedy is given to patients in this category it will act as though it were a constitutional remedy, i.e. the whole person will improve.

In other cases the disorder is more general, but there exists a weak link in the chain and it is often advantageous to strengthen this before giving constitutional treatment. Whether the organ weakness is considered primary or not, the past medical history together with the symptoms and observable signs should all be used as pointers to determine the affected organs.

Generally speaking, the majority of patients who benefit from organ remedies will still require constitutional, miasmatic or other more generalised treatment in order to be fully and permanently cured.

Reducing Aggravations

I am convinced that many of the aggravations which occur following constitutional prescriptions can be lessened or avoided altogether by the judicious application of organ support remedies. Hahnemann taught that the curative process should be rapid, permanent and *gentle*, whereas some of the responses I have seen following a high potency constitutional prescription have been anything except gentle.

Patients aggravate for different reasons and in different ways, but a good many aggravations result when the indicated constitutional remedy that is prescribed has a strong affinity for the patient's weakest organ. For example, *Kali carbonicum* or *Lycopodium* is given where the liver is weak, *Aurum* or *Tuberculinum* where the heart is weak, *Sulphur* (in skin cases especially) where the eliminative organs are underfunctioning, etc. Many of these types of aggravation will occur even using a low potency of the indicated remedy, and they are mostly predictable and preventable. All that is necessary is to determine the weakest organ before giving the constitutional remedy and to 'tone it up' using an appropriate support remedy. This will usually be accomplished within a month or two, after which the constitutional remedy may be given with impunity in whatever potency is desired.

Advantages of Organ Supports

I have heard practitioners state that to give an organ support remedy which is not indicated constitutionally is suppressive and will do harm to the patient. Anyone who has used organ remedies extensively will know that this is nonsense. One of the commonest responses my patients have reported after a course of organ support treatment is that they feel better in themselves - and this is *before* they have been given any constitutional treatment! Sometimes the general improvement can be quite staggering.

A further benefit I have observed is that the constitutional remedy picture often becomes sharper and more clearly defined. When energy is no longer being diverted to sustaining a sluggish organ, that is what I would expect to happen, and I have seen it many times. Sometimes I have been undecided between several constitutional remedies, each seeming equally well indicated, yet after prescribing an organ remedy the constitutional picture has become blatantly obvious.

Case Examples

Case One

A man in his thirties suffered with persistent wheezing for over four years, having started shortly before his first child was due to be born. His breathing was worse in the evenings, and much worse after alcohol, and he was using Ventolin & Becotide inhalers daily. He had recurrent sinus infections; a tendency to thick, yellow mucus in his nose and throat, this also was worse in the evenings and after alcohol. He had very low energy, especially between 3 and 5pm; he felt shattered on awaking. He craved sweets; liked rich and fried foods but found they disagreed with him. His bowels became loose when nervous, e.g. before an exam. He was sensitive to the cold, with very cold feet, especially at night. His teeth were yellow, he had a sallow complexion, dark rings around his eyes and he looked exhausted. His tongue was coated whitish-yellow. At 18 years of age he had suffered glandular fever which lasted for three months and took him twelve months to recover from.

If this patient had been treated constitutionally he would have been given *Lycopodium*, which was indicated both mentally and generally. Paying attention to the signs and symptoms, it was clear to me that his liver was his weakest organ. All of the following, when taken collectively, point to a weakness of the liver:

Aggravation fats; rich food; alcohol
Low energy in general; on waking; between 3pm and 5pm
Yellow complexion; catarrh; tongue
Cold extremities
Craves sweets
History of prolonged glandular fever

Initially he was given *Carcinosin* 30, 200, 1M on the history of severe glandular fever and the family history. This increased the production of mucus from his sinuses and his energy improved slightly. Apart from that there was little other response.

I then prescribed for him *Chelidonium* fluid extract, 2 drops in water t.d.s. and suggested he avoided using the inhalers as much as possible. Firstly he developed a foul taste in his mouth which lasted for several days; then he noticed his sinuses clearing and his sense of smell becoming stronger. His energy increased considerably and the wheeziness disappeared, despite his having abandoned the inhalers. His complexion improved dramatically, he felt 'more alive' on awaking and found that his feet became warm, even at night. His axillary glands became swollen and tender for several days (an old symptom) and then returned to normal. All of this occurred in the space of four weeks on the organ remedy, and constitutional treatment had yet to begin. He was subsequently given *Lycopodium* 1M with further improvement and only slight aggravation. My guess is that had *Lycopodium* been given as a first prescription he would have suffered considerably from the response to it.

I have found that a support remedy for the liver is beneficial in an astonishing number of cases, particularly when you find a history of jaundice, gall-bladder trouble, alcohol abuse, hepatitis or glandular fever. Sometimes glandular fever will leave a residual weakness in the spleen rather than the liver, and *Ceanothus* is a wonderful remedy in these cases.

Case Two

I treated a 59 year old woman who complained of a hiatus hernia which had troubled her for years. She regurgitated food at least four times and up to six times in a day, aggravated if she bent forward at all. Sometimes she would bring up a greasy watery fluid. She had burning in her stomach and rising upwards, and an acidic taste in her mouth. She was overweight, had very low energy and became breathless on slight exertion. She suffered palpitations on exertion or bending. She became hot and sweated easily, but suffered with cold feet. Her hands and ankles became very swollen during the day. She was fearful of the dark and had a fear of cancer.

My initial impression was that this patient needed *Calcarea carbonica* as a constitutional remedy, and that the digestive tract was the focus of the case. However, I noticed that she had a staring, almost exophthalmic look which one would normally associate with hyperthyroidism - despite her other symptoms pointing to *hypo*-thyroidism if anything. Intrigued, I palpated her thyroid and found it normal. Furthermore, she suggested I didn't waste my time with this because she had had blood tests recently and her thyroid activity was deemed to be normal. Still not convinced, I decided to follow one of Burnett's suggestions. He said that sometimes the only reliable way to confirm an organ-diagnosis was to give an organ remedy and to see whether it acted.

Knowing it had a reputation as a regulator of thyroid function, I prescribed *Fucus vesiculosus* 3x, one tablet to be taken q.d. After two weeks treatment she reported having gone four whole days without regurgitating her food once! She felt better in herself, her urinary output had increased, her hands and ankles were less swollen and she was sure she was losing weight. After a few weeks more she had shed several pounds, with further improvement in the digestive symptoms. I continued *Fucus* until it seemed to do no more for her, and then gave her *Calcarea carbonica* 10M and it seemed to pick up the work where *Fucus* had left off. Over the course of three and a half months treatment she lost 15lbs in weight without any change in her diet or lifestyle.

This was the sort of case where it definitely paid off to give the organ remedy before starting the constitutional treatment. Had I prescribed *Calcarea* from the outset together with *Fucus*, the constitutional remedy would undoubtedly have been given the credit for the response. The only conclusion I could draw about the hiatus hernia was that it must have been secondary to her obesity, which in turn was secondary to a thyroid imbalance. All of this proves the point that Rademacher made about treating the *primary* organ disease, which may be quite remote from where the symptoms are manifesting.

Further reading:
M. Wood
The Book of Herbal Wisdom - Using Plants as Medicines
North Atlantic Books

Rademacher's Universal and Organ Remedies
Translated by A.A. Ramseyer
A.P. Homeo Library, Calcutta-700001, India

J. Compton Burnett
The Best of Burnett
Jain Publishing Co., New Delhi, India

Yadubir Sinha
Miracles of Mother Tinctures
World Homeopathic Links, New Delhi-110055, India
Jacques Jouanny
The Essentials of Homeopathic Therapeutics
Laboratoires Boiron, Lyon, France

Y.R. Agrawal
Materia Medica of Glandular Medicines
Vijay Publications, Delhi-110092, India

K. Kansal
Handbook of Homeopathic Mother Tinctures
Pratap Medical Publishers, New Delhi, India

E.A. Maury
Drainage in Homeopathy (Detoxification)
C.W. Daniel Co. Ltd., Saffron Walden, Essex

I. Watson
Organ Remedies
Seven Herbs
Recorded Seminars, available in Audiotape and CD formats
www.ianwatsonseminars.com

Physical Generals

Definition
This is a variation on constitutional treatment, differing only in that physical general symptoms are graded highest in the hierarchy of symptoms, above mental/emotional and physical particular symptoms. By physical general is meant any physical symptom or modality which refers to the patient as a whole and not just to one part.

Background
Boenninghausen (1785-1864), working before the advent of psychotherapy, drew attention to the importance of general symptoms over particulars, and constructed his *Therapeutic Pocket Book* to reflect this approach. It is worth noting that Kent also laid emphasis on the physical general symptoms. In his article entitled *How to Use the Repertory[1]*, Kent states quite clearly that for purposes of repertorisation he prefers to take the general symptoms and modalities *first*, followed by the emotional and intellectual symptoms.

It was C. M. Boger (1861-1935) who was able to synthesize the teachings of both Boenninghausen and Kent, and thereby refine and extend the physical generals approach. The outcome of this was a much-enlarged edition of Boennninghausen's original work, entitled *Boenninghausen's Characteristics and Repertory*, and later came the compact yet highly comprehensive *Synoptic Key of the Materia Medica*. This latter work is truly a goldmine for those who will take the trouble to study it in depth.

Phatak's Repertory
Phatak's *Concise Repertory* was first published in 1963 and is therefore one of the most recent of all the repertories. I have found in practice that it is the ideal tool to use when the generals are taken to form the basis for the prescription. This repertory contains rubrics for many general symptoms and states which are not adequately represented in Kent's *Repertory*, nor anywhere else. It is an extension of the work begun by Boger called the *Supplemental Reference Table* which is located at the back of his *Synoptic Key of the Materia Medica*. The repertory is laid out alphabetically rather than schematically, so that once the reader is familiar with the contents it is extremely easy to use.

Examples of general rubrics from Phatak's Repertory
Below are examples of some of the general rubrics to be found in Phatak's *Repertory*. It will be noted that very often a single rubric encompasses several

related states, for which a series of smaller, separate rubrics would have to be consulted in the larger repertories. Once the idea of generalising symptoms is grasped, the process of repertorisation becomes much less mechanical and time-consuming and allows for greater creativity on the part of the practitioner.

Alternating effects, states, sides, metastasis
Ball, lump, knot etc.
Bluish, purple (discharges, discoloration of skin etc.)
Children, infants
Chronicity
Desquamation, branny, scaly etc.
Duality, in pieces, separated, as if someone else
Enlarged, swelled, as if
Females, affections of
Fishy, odour, taste etc.
Growth affected, disorders of
Heaviness, load
Loose, as if
Lumps, lumpy effects
Nutrition affected
Pregnancy, Childbed, affections of, or since Agg.
Puberty, affections of
Relapses, recurrences
Salty, saltiness
Wooden feeling
Yellowness (of skin, discharges etc)

Advantages of the Generals Approach
The main advantage of this method is that far less psychological interpretation is required on the part of the practitioner in order to arrive at the indicated remedy. Interestingly, I have often found that a remedy worked out in this way is later discovered to cover very fundamental psychological symptoms in the case which were either missed or misinterpreted by the practitioner or withheld by the patient. Not having been trained in psycho-analysis, I prefer to let the physical body guide me to the constitutional remedy whenever I am at all doubtful of the psychological component, and this is fairly often. To me, this is one of the beauties of homeopathy - that the wheel has many spokes, all leading to the same centre. There is no need to dogmatically stick to one route when the patient is telling you quite blatantly that another, more reliable path is available to you.

Another advantage of this method is that the remedies which are considered "difficult to perceive" by prescribers who rely primarily on the psyche of the patient become just as easy to perceive as any other remedy. Examples would be *Thuja, Mercurius & Kali carbonicum,* all of which I was taught are difficult remedies to pin down due to the psychological natures of the individuals needing them. I find in practice that I arrive at these remedies as often as any other, almost always by means of characteristic symptoms or the physical generals method, ignoring any dubious mentals.

Types of General Symptoms
Below are some of the major categories of physical general symptoms with which the prescriber should be familiar. Boger always emphasised the *modalities* especially, because they require the least interpretation of all - if asthmatic breathing is relieved by bending forward, then that is so and nobody can be in any doubt about it. Of all the modalities, he stressed the *time of aggravation* as being especially noteworthy, because it is often the least explainable from a pathological point of view, and is therefore characteristic of the patient.

Modalities: times of day or night; periodicity; temperature; weather; seasons; moon phases; position; motion; rest; touch; pressure etc.

Sensations: heat or chilliness; throbbing; cutting; burning; sore, bruised; cramping; smarting; stitching etc.

Localities: sides of body; direction and alternation of sides; organs and tissues affected; extension of pain or sensation to other parts.

Observable signs: facial expression; demeanour; excitability; restlessness; apathy; colour and nature of discharges & secretions; colour and texture of skin etc.

Aetiologies: never been well since......... grief; anger; bad news; vaccination; suppressed eruptions; injury; puberty; childbirth; menopause etc.

Food: cravings; strong aversions; aggravations; alterations of thirst. Particularly important when these have changed or become intensified since the patient became ill, for example, "I used to crave sweet things, but now I find I dislike them".

Menses: early; late; absent; scanty; profuse; clotted; bright; dark; painful;

ailments before, during or after.

Sexual desire & function: increased; diminished; absent; perverted; suppressed.

Generalising Particulars
When a patient suffers the same kind of symptom in several different parts, these particular symptoms can often be grouped together to form a physical general, which is of higher prescribing value than each of the particulars taken separately. This approach was developed originally by Boeninghausen and later taken up by Boger.

As an example, a patient may complain of right-sided headaches, rheumatism worse on the right side and a tendency to pains in the right kidney region. In this patient 'right sided' is a general symptom, and it is very likely a remedy is needed that has a strong affinity for the right side, such as *Lycopodium*.

In chronic cases, generalisation of particulars can be taken a stage further by identifying the common thread that often runs through the whole history of a person's health problems. For example, a patient may present with menopausal flushes and congestive, throbbing headaches. The history reveals that her menstrual periods always used to be heavy with throbbing pains on the first day. Twenty years ago she had gall-stone colic with hot, throbbing pains. In this case the sensation 'throbbing' is a general symptom and a remedy that didn't cover this would be unlikely to be deeply curative.

Defective Cases
There is a category of cases which, from a prescribing point of view, remain incomplete or defective in some way or another despite careful efforts to complete the case. There are also chronic cases that produce confusion because they contain several seemingly independent groups of symptoms all calling for attention and yet failing to fall into a single cohesive pattern. In attempting to unravel these types of case, Boeninnghausen had the idea that as every local symptom was but a reflection of a greater whole, then it should be possible to construct a picture of the totality by analogy from details of the fragmented parts.

For example, supposing a patient complained of headaches, a skin eruption and joint problems. It is possible that there might be a common thread which connects all of these complaints, for instance they might all be aggravated by heat. But equally, they may all appear to have differing modalities and sensations, so a different approach is needed. What Boenninghausen discovered is that it is possible to make sense of a case like this by selecting a single, outstanding factor from each different area and bringing them all together for analysis.

First he might obtain a definite location or problem area - say for instance *Joints and Skin*. Then he would obtain a definite sensation - suppose that the headaches were throbbing, he would take the general sensation *Throbbing*. Then he would find a strong modality - suppose that both the joints and the headaches were relieved by pressure, he would take the general modality *Better for Pressure*. Then, to complete the picture he would look for a concomitant symptom, that is, something occurring outside of the main symptom groups. Suppose for example the patient was highly anxious, he might take *Anxiety* as a general concomitant.

The structure of the case now ready to be repertorised is as follows:

Joints & Skin
Throbbing
> Pressure
Anxiety

This symptom-group can now be taken to contain a representative sample of the patient as a whole, and can therefore be repertorised using the *general* rubrics in the repertory rather than the particulars.

In certain cases, it is only the particular (local) symptoms that express clear modalities, sensations etc., therefore these must be utilised but they can be taken to be representative of the general state and repertorised using general rubrics.

Case Example
A woman complained of dermatitis of the hands which became worse before each menstrual period. It had pronounced itching, aggravated by getting the hands wet. Whilst she had the condition previously, it had become much worse following the birth of her son.

In this case the general symptoms were very well defined, whereas the particular (skin) symptoms were quite clear. Taking these to be a reflection of her general state, I repertorised the case using Phatak's *Repertory* and choosing the following *general* rubrics:

Skin affections, Menses Agg. (p. 310)
Menses, Before Agg. (p. 229)
Bathing, Aversion to or Agg. (p. 30)
Pregnancy, Childbed, Affections of, or Since Agg. (p. 276)

The remedy that came through was *Sepia*, and this was given in the 12th potency with the result that she improved generally and the dermatitis became milder and became confined to the fingers only, showing the proper direction of cure. She was subsequently given *Bovista* and later *Natrum muriaticum* which completed the cure. This case demonstrates how, as Boenninghausen suggested, the modalities of particular symptoms can indeed be 'generalised' to good effect. I would especially recommend this technique in cases where the *particular* symptoms predominate, but a prescription based on these exclusively fails to act or is only palliative, as is often the case.

Prescribing Technique
The prescribing guidelines to be found under the chapter on Constitutional Prescribing apply equally to this method. One of the keys to success with the Physical Generals method is only to utilise the *outstanding* symptoms in the case, in whatever category. This is important because the rubrics in Phatak's *Concise Repertory* only contain those remedies that are known to have the corresponding symptom or state markedly. Therefore, in order to succeed with the method requires the prescriber to select the symptoms that are strong in the patient and match these to a remedy that has those symptoms in equal strength. Numerous vague, common or dubious symptoms should always be ignored in preference to a few strong, clear and prominent ones.

Prescribing on the physical generals often requires a right-brain approach to case analysis, as the prescriber is encouraged to make connections between isolated symptoms, to synthesize rather than particularise.

When to Use the Method
In any case where a constitutional prescription is sought but where the mental/emotional symptoms are either withheld or are too vague, too deficient or too common to prescribe on, then the physical generals approach will prove invaluable. Similarly in cases which are considered incomplete or confused, this technique can allow the whole person still to be treated rather than the parts.
This method can also be extremely helpful in cases where only partially-similar remedies can be found by any method, and the deeper curative action desired cannot be achieved. I have often combed through all the notes gathered from a series of consultations and put together all the general symptoms that have

been present at one time or another, then repertorised the resulting group. I have noticed when doing this that often the patient has expressed the same idea in slightly different ways on separate occasions, thus it seemed as though they were different symptoms when in fact they are all one and the same. This approach often throws up remedies that hadn't previously been considered for the case, or had been rejected because they didn't appear to match a mental or perhaps a particular symptom.

Case Example

A woman complained of premenstrual syndrome of many years duration, which acupuncture and previous homeopathic treatment had only palliated. Before each period for at least one week she suffered with aching pains in the legs, worse on lying down; insomnia, waking around 3am and unable to get back to sleep; great exhaustion; emotional instability with frequent changes of mood. Her periods came at intervals of three weeks.

She had a tendency to recurrent backache in the lumbar region, since giving birth fifteen years previously. History of post-natal depression lasting many months. She had two children and had difficulties during both pregnancies; the first birth was a forceps delivery. She was generally chilly. Sweated easily, especially at night in bed. Recurrent sore, bruised pain in the region of the liver with occasional sharp stitches. Sleepiness after her evening meal. Stools tended to be very pale.

This case presented clear physical generals but a deficiency of pronounced mental or emotional symptoms, and was therefore ideally suited to the physical generals method. I repertorised the case using Phatak's *Repertory*, taking the following rubrics:

Menses, Before Agg. (p. 229)
Menses, Early (p. 232)
Pregnancy, Childbed, affections of, or since Agg. (p 276)
Liver (& right hypochondria) (p. 217)
Time, 3am Agg. (p. 360)
Changing Moods (p. 46)

Because so many of her sufferings were worse before the period, to save time I used the rubric 'Menses, before Agg.' as an eliminator, that is to say I only considered the remedies in that rubric. Whilst *Cocculus* and *Calcarea Carbonica* featured strongly in the repertorisation, *Kali carbonicum* was the only remedy to be found in every rubric. Seeing that it matched the emphasis of the case very well, I prescribed a single dose of *Kali carb.* 30.

The result was an aggravation of her symptoms lasting almost five weeks, during which time several old symptoms returned and subsequently disappeared. After this she suddenly started to improve and her periods then established a four-weekly cycle and she had none of the premenstrual symptoms. The improvement lasted for three months, after which a return of some of the cured symptoms called for a repetition. *Kali carb.* 200 was given, which produced another lengthy but less intense aggravation and she then remained well for almost a year, when a further dose was needed.

The curative action of the remedy in this case was very deep and it was obviously a remedy that she had needed for many years. With hindsight, I am sure that an organ support remedy for the liver prescribed before the *Kali carb.* would have considerably lessened the extent of the aggravations she suffered (see Organ Remedies).

Further Reading

C. M. Boger
A Synoptic Key of the Materia Medica
Boenninghausen's Characteristics and Repertory
Jain Publishing Co., New Delhi, India
Studies in the Philosophy of Healing
World Homeopathic Links, New Delhi, India

S. R. Phatak
A Concise Repertory of Homeopathic Medicines
Homeopathic Medical Publishers, Bombay, India

H. A. Roberts
The Principles and Practicability of Boenninghausen's Therapeutic Pocket Book
Jain Publishing Co., New Delhi, India

P. Sankaran
Introduction to Boger's Synoptic Key
Homeopathic Medical Publishers, Bombay, India

Polypharmacy

Definition

This method encompasses any prescribing technique in which two or more remedies are prescribed *simultaneously*, either in alternation with each other or as a combined formula.

Prescribing Technique

Polypharmacy may be *individualised*, whereby several remedies are given concurrently or alternately according to indications in each individual case. It may also be *disease-based*, whereby multiple remedies are prescribed solely on the basis that they all have a degree of similarity to a particular disease process, without due regard for individual peculiarities (e.g. Nelsons' combination remedy for hay fever).

Generally low potencies are more frequently employed, mostly within the range Ø - 6c, and the prescription is repeated usually on a daily basis. I find that the biochemic tissue salts are ideally suited to this method, and prefer to combine the appropriate single remedies to suit the patient rather than rely on the commercially-available compound formulæ.

Individualised Polypharmacy

As with homeopathy generally, my own experience with polypharmacy has been that better results are obtained the more the prescription is tailored to suit the individual patient.

One of the past masters of individualised polypharmacy was undoubtedly J. Ellis Barker, a journalist turned homeopath who practised widely and wrote extensively in the 1930's and 40's. Two of his best works are modestly entitled *New Lives for Old - How to Cure the Incurable* and *Miracles of Healing and How They are Done.* Barker was well-versed in dietary and other naturopathic techniques and he received his homeopathic inspiration from the great J. H. Clarke. His resulting style of practice was unashamedly eclectic, as had been Clarke's, and the only justification that mattered to him was that he obtained curative results with his methods, often in apparently hopeless cases.

I learnt a great deal from studying Ellis Barker's writings. Apart from anything else, he certainly knew how to *enthuse* his patients into getting well, which isn't widely taught to students of homeopathy these days.

Ellis Barker's system seemed to operate as follows: *if you see an indication for a remedy, you give it, sooner rather than later.* So, for example, if a patient presented to him with chronic constipation, indigestion and flatulence, a history of adverse reaction to vaccination and a tubercular family history, the first prescription would typically be as follows:

Carbo veg. 6x twice daily in alternation with *Nux vomica* 6x twice daily; *Thuja* 30 each Saturday and *Bacillinum* 200 each Wednesday.

Barker obtained impressive results with his method and he had little time for those who would rather stick to their principles and let their patients suffer than treat them differently and get them better.

The French homeopath Jacques Jouanny has developed an all-embracing system of multiple-remedy prescribing which has much in common with Ellis Barker's method. In chronic cases he advocates giving the basic constitutional remedy of the patient together with an intercurrent miasmatic nosode, plus one or more low potency remedies for the disorder. I have absolutely no reason to doubt that he obtains curative results in this way.

It is interesting to note that despite his public admonitions to the contrary, privately Hahnemann was not averse to prescribing several remedies simultaneously or in alternation with one another, as recent translations of his casenotes[1] have revealed. Being the great experimenter that he was, it is hardly surprising that he should do so. The argument that polypharmacy is anti-Hahnemannian has little basis in fact.

Non-individualised Polypharmacy

For as long as homeopathy has existed, the temptation to combine several remedies together and prescribe them for a specific disease has been too great to resist. The theoretical advantage is that by combining say, five of the most commonly prescribed remedies for earache, the practitioner is able to bypass the necessity to individualise each case and give every earache patient the same prescription. The assumption is either that whichever remedy in the combination is most similar to the earache of the person being treated will act and the other, non-indicated remedies will do nothing, or that a group of remedies known to bear similarity to the typical symptoms of earache will, collectively, bring about a curative response.

I have tried many of the disease orientated combination formulæ for problems such as hay fever, catarrh, pain, varicose veins and so on, and generally the results have been disappointing, with a few notable successes. As far as I can ascertain, when prescribed routinely these combinations seem to work palliatively or not at all in a fairly high percentage of cases, and curatively in a smaller number. For this reason I would prefer to prescribe a single remedy or prepare a multiple prescription on an individualised basis wherever possible, as the results seem to justify the extra effort required.

A combination remedy of which I am unaware of the origin but which seems to be widely recommended is the following:

Sulphur 6x
Silica 6x
Carbo veg. 6x

This remedy is known by its abbreviation *S.S.C.* and is indicated for adolescent acne and as a general 'cleanser of the blood'.

The late Thomas Maughan, upon whose original teachings much of the current homeopathic training in the U.K. is based, developed a range of combination remedies from his own experience. Like the above, they mostly comprise three remedies combined together in tincture or low potency, and some of the indications for their use are extremely precise. As far as I am aware these combinations have never been published, the originator having preferred to pass his wisdom on by apprenticeship and direct teaching, and I suspect they are not widely used today.

One of Thomas Maughan's combinations which I have used successfully is:

Arnica 6x (1 part)
Cratægus Ø (2 parts)
Kali mur. 3x (1 part)

This combination is indicated for post-apoplectic patients, to promote reabsorption of the clot, reduce the tendency to further strokes and to deal with any resulting weakness in the heart and arteries. I once gave this prescription to an elderly Indian gentleman who had suffered a major stroke and he amazed everyone (including me) with the speed and extent of his recovery.

Another of his better known combinations is known as the 'peace of mind pill' and contains the following:

Ambra grisea 6x
Anacardium 6x
Argentum nit. 6x

This remedy is to help those suffering in anticipation of some ordeal, or who are troubled and worried over many things.

Clarke recommends polypharmacy in his writings for certain cases, particularly of acute disease. For example, in his Dictionary[2] he suggests *Morbillinum* be given in alternation with *Belladonna* in cases of measles. In The Prescriber[3] he advocates giving *Coqueluchinum* (his own preparation of *Pertussin*) in alternation with 'some other well-indicated remedy' in whooping cough. He also recommends combining *Bacillinum* 30 with *Influenzinum* 30, this to be given once weekly as a prophylactic during influenza epidemics. I have used this latter combination in elderly patients for whom a dose of 'flu is generally worth avoiding, and it seems to be effective as a prophylactic given at fortnightly or monthly intervals throughout the winter.

Case example
A woman in her eighties had suffered several heart attacks and now complained of vertigo, joint problems, dyspnoea, lethargy, chest pains, fluid retention, itching skin, constipation and insomnia.

She was treated constitutionally first of all, with *Calcarea carbonica* and later *Arsenicum*. I also tried *Cratægus* Ø as an organ support remedy for her weak heart. This approach achieved little other than aggravation of her symptoms and left her even more listless and despondent than before. Having watched her endure several months of this without relief, in desperation I prescribed the following recipe:

Diphtherinum 30 each Wednesday (on a history of diphtheria badly when younger)
Psorinum 30 each Saturday (on the miasmatic background)
P36* t.d.s. after meals

*P36 is one of many combination remedies formulated by E. F. W. Powell for the supportive treatment of different conditions. This particular combination comprises:
Calc fluor. 8x
Kali phos. 6x
Ferrum phos. 6x

Digitalis 6x
Convallaria 3x
Crataegus 3x
Cactus 3x

It is indicated for heart weakness and valvular trouble.

After three weeks treatment she returned and said: "I feel more alive." Her energy and motivation were markedly improved, her breathing was easier and the chest pains were better. The itching had started to subside and her sleep was improved. Understandably, she wanted to know why I hadn't given her that prescription in the first place!

The Arguments Against

There are two main arguments against polypharmacy that have any validity. The first is that as our remedies were proven singly, they ought only to be given singly, as no-one can predict how several remedies will act on an individual when given simultaneously. The implication here is that untold misery and suffering may result from such a deviation from traditional methods. This is theoretically sound, but in practice the fears turn out to be unfounded, as anyone who has given polypharmacy a fair trial will testify. The worse that I have seen happen after a combined prescription has been that the patient didn't get better, which I have also seen many times following the administration of a single remedy.

The second argument is that the practitioner will be uncertain as to which remedy worked, assuming a curative response takes place at all. This I acknowledge to be a frustration sometimes, mostly because a learning opportunity has been missed, but it should be noted that this is something which bothers practitioners, not patients. Most of my patients couldn't care less whether I prescribe one remedy or six, as long as they get better.

When to Use the Method

I find that polypharmacy is best suited to serious cases, particularly where disease is manifesting in several different ways simultaneously, and to cases in which palliation is more desirable or more likely than cure. I am sure that in certain cases polypharmacy will achieve the desired result in a shorter period of time than would have been the case using single remedies, which is no doubt why Clarke recommended it for cutting short acute diseases. However, I will generally use a single-remedy approach first wherever possible, the main reason being that this affords the best opportunity for learning about the action of remedies. If I knew in advance which patients would do better on polypharmacy then I would give it to them first without any hesitation.

Further Reading
Ellis Barker, J.
Miracles of Healing and How they are done
How to Cure the Incurable
Jain Publications, New Delhi, India

Jouanny, Jacques
The Essentials of Homeopathic Therapeutics
Translated from the French by D. Clausen
Laboratoires Boiron, France

Powell, Eric F.W.
The Group Remedy Prescriber
Martin and Pleasance Wholesale, Victoria, Australia

Repertorisation

The best repertory any one can have is in his own memory

John H. Clarke
The Prescriber

Definition

Repertory = index, list, catalogue

This method embraces a variety of techniques whereby a repertory is employed to determine a small group of remedies, from which the most similar one to the case may be chosen.

Introduction

Repertories were introduced into homeopathy because the expanding materia medica became, even in Hahnemann's lifetime, too voluminous to allow quick and easy reference. A repertory provides an efficient means of accessing the materia medica, without having to read and compare endless lists of symptoms. The purpose of repertorisation, however, is not to replace materia medica study. Rather it is designed to provide a bridge between the case being worked on and the remedy pictures in the materia medica. A successful repertorisation takes the prescriber to those few remedies bearing close similarity to the case, which may then be studied and compared in the materia medica to determine the final choice. Some practitioners are highly skilled in the use of a repertory and are able, by selecting the rubrics very carefully, to narrow the choice down to one remedy using the repertory alone.

The most important thing to keep in mind is that a repertory should be considered as a complement to, not a replacement for the materia medica. Those practitioners I have met who are repertory technicians of the highest order are first and foremost, without exception, masters of the materia medica.

Repertories in Use

Kent's *Repertory* has dominated the scene for the best part of the last century. Kent is said to have laboured for over sixteen years to produce it, and many homeopaths still rank it as one of the standard works of reference. It is, however, seriously outdated now in its original form, so thankfully there have been numerous attempts to update, revise and replace it.

The *Synthetic Repertory* of Barthel and Klunker is basically an updated version

82

of Kent's *Repertory*, with additional material from a wide variety of sources. This repertory is produced in three volumes, but unfortunately contains no particular symptoms whatsoever. Other modern repertories following the same format as Kent but with much additional material have been produced by Eizayaga and Kunzli. Yet another modern repertory based on Kent's which has gained a strong following amongst classical homeopaths is the *Synthesis Repertory* of Ed. F. Schroyens. Containing around 200,000 additions to Kent's original version and based on the *RADAR* computer repertory programme, this is probably the best Kentian-style repertory currently available in book form. Another Kentian repertory which is not for the faint-hearted is the *Complete Repertory* of R. Van-Zandvoort, based upon the *MacRepertory* computer programme.

Robin Murphy's *Homeopathic Medical Repertory* is, for me, the most user-friendly and versatile repertory currently available. It was first published in 1993 and was quickly sold out and replaced by a considerably revised second edition. The format has been a source of some controversy, as Murphy took the radical step of replacing the Kentian schema with a completely alphabetical layout. Whilst it takes a bit of getting used to for those raised on Kent, it is in my experience much quicker and easier to access once you are familiar with it. Those who have never been exposed to a Kentian-style repertory should, in my opinion, save themselves a huge amount of unnecessary labour and simply start off with this one.

Another criticism levelled at Murphy is that his repertory lacks the references scattered throughout repertories such as Kunzli's, which enable the user to trace the source of remedy and rubric additions. Personally I find these references superfluous, and Kent himself never saw the need to include them. To me, a repertory will always be a dynamic, imperfect and incomplete reference work, and I feel that any homeopath's clinical experience is as valid as anybody else's. There is a kind of elitism within homeopathy these days which suggests that certain 'masters' are to be trusted, and clinical experiences coming from any other source must be treated with suspicion - a delusion of superiority if ever there was one!

Although there are more comprehensive repertories available now, Murphy's has several key features that make it a favourite amongst thousands of users worldwide. Apart from the alphabetical format, it also contains a large number of clinical rubrics and modern-day terms such as such as *Raynaud's Disease, Allergic Reactions, Multiple Sclerosis, Endometriosis, Chemotherapy agg.,* etc. Murphy's repertory also has some wonderful new chapters which gather together a mountain of information scattered throughout the homeopathic literature. These include *Environment, Food, Blood, Children, Diseases, Toxicity* and *Emergencies.*

Phatak's *Concise Repertory* is still one of my favourite homeopathic books, and is especially useful when using the physical generals approach. I find Phatak's *Repertory* to be a wonderful time-saver in practice provided it is used appropriately and within its limitations. If there are mental or particular symptoms to be repertorised, Murphy is usually a better choice. To save time, I will often select a single general rubric from Phatak to start an elimination repertorisation (see below), and then use rubrics from Murphy for the remainder.

Boenninghausen's *Characteristics and Repertory* is one of the earliest repertories, but was completely revised and updated by Boger in the early part of this century. It is a major work, but is probably doomed to stay on the back shelves of most homeopathic libraries these days.

Clarke's *Clinical Repertory* was produced as a companion volume to his *Dictionary of Materia Medica* and *The Prescriber,* with which it is cross-referenced to some extent. It actually contains four repertories in one, as it includes sections on causations, temperaments and relationships of remedies as well as the clinical index. Its main advantage is that it tends to emphasise the minor remedies, whereas virtually every other repertory tends to emphasise the polychrests. However, this is offset by the fact that Clarke chose to use different remedy abbreviations to every other author, which renders it somewhat confusing to use.

There are literally dozens of 'lesser' repertories available, most of which focus on a particular disease state or bring together data from many sources on a similar theme, such as causation, dreams, time aggravations etc. One such repertory I have found helpful is the *Homeopathic Aide-Memoire* written by Peter Coats. This is essentially a pocket-sized repertory for acute prescribing, but contains other gems of clinical information as well.

When to Repertorise
Repertorisation can be used to support almost any prescribing technique, but it is probably most effectively used when symptom-similarity is the primary basis for the prescription, the reason being that the repertories we have available are chiefly composed of symptom-lists. It is generally less appropriate when using a miasmatic or organopathic approach. Some repertories, such as Clarke's and

Murphy's are more clinically orientated and are therefore useful in supporting a therapeutics approach.

Repertorisation Techniques
There are three main ways in which a repertory may be used in practice:

1) Spot Checking
This means simply flicking through the repertory to find a key rubric in the case and noting which remedies feature. Many practitioners do this during the case-taking as a means of checking out a particular line of enquiry, eliminating or confirming a remedy or group of remedies in mind.

Case Example
A twelve year-old boy was brought into our clinic displaying behavioural problems and various digestive disturbances. *Lycopodium* seemed well-indicated for him but had failed to make much impression, so we questioned him further. Asked about fears, he reflected a little, then responded without any shadow of doubt that he had a fear of being paralyzed! Not knowing if such a symptom even existed in the materia medica, I went straight to Kent's *Repertory* where the symptom was found in the Mind section with just five remedies listed. The only remedy in italics was *Anacardium*, which was found to cover the rest of the case well and was given with marked improvement. This case demonstrates the value of a spot-check and illustrates how rapid a repertorisation can be, provided the characteristic symptoms are chosen at the outset.

2) Elimination Repertorisation
This is a more thorough technique but is designed to prevent the prescriber having to write out lengthy lists of remedies, most of which need not be considered. The method involves choosing a key symptom from the case about which it can be said that *the remedy the patient needs has to be in the corresponding rubric*. That primary rubric is then taken as a starting point, and only the remedies listed in it are repertorised any further. There are several instances in which this is an appropriate strategy:

i) When there is a clearcut, direct aetiology in the case (see Aetiologies). For example, if someone dates all of their presenting complaints back to a severe fright, 'ailments from fright' may be taken as the primary rubric. It is very unlikely that a remedy outside of that group will be needed.

It is worth noting that in the *Synthetic Repertory* all of the ætiological rubrics which are scattered throughout the mind section of Kent's *Repertory* have been brought together under the single heading *'Ailments from'*.

ii) When there exists a single, *outstanding* symptom in the case, in any category (mental, emotional or physical; general or particular), provided it has an unusual intensity, peculiarity or uniqueness in the type of case being treated (see Symptoms). As an example, I treated a woman with a degenerative nervous system disease whose sufferings were always aggravated at the full moon. I took the rubric *'Moon Phases, Full Moon etc. Agg.'* (Phatak's *Repertory,* page 237) as an eliminator, which, although it contains only a small number of remedies, was a safe choice because of the peculiarity of the modality. The rest of the case repertorised out to *Alumina,* which was given with great benefit.

iii) When there exists a clearly-defined pathological process, provided no other outstanding feature of the case exists to over-ride this. For example, if the patient clearly has cancer or measles or hepatitis, the corresponding rubric may be safely chosen for elimination purposes *unless* there is a symptom in the case which is so strong or peculiar as to take precedence. It should be remembered that if the disease is to be treated first, only those symptoms that pertain to the disease should be included in the repertorisation.

Supposing a child is brought in with measles, the rubric *'Fevers, measles'* from Murphy can be used as a safe starting point in the vast majority of cases. The other symptoms of the case may then be used to narrow down that group, but any symptoms which existed *before* the measles and which are unchanged should not be included. If, for example, the child has had a great thirst since the onset of the measles, then it is a symptom of the disease and should be repertorised. If, however, the child has *always* been that thirsty, then it is a symptom of the person and should only be repertorised when treating constitutionally, *after* the measles has been cured.

3) Totality Repertorisation
Unless a computer is employed, this is the most cumbersome of all repertory techniques, and it should therefore be reserved for those cases where another technique cannot be used and/or where time is available in abundance. All of the symptoms considered to be important are located in the repertory and every complete rubric is copied out in full. The whole group of rubrics is then analysed to see which remedies feature in most or all of the rubrics. This type of repertorisation produces two things: firstly it may be seen which remedies appear in the most rubrics (a purely *quantitative* analysis), and secondly each remedy may be given a 'score' by adding together all of the grades of type

in which it appears (a more *qualitative* analysis). Using Murphy's or Kent's *Repertory* for instance, remedies appearing in **bold type** will score three, those in *italics* will score two and those in ordinary type will score one.

The end result of a totality repertorisation is a small group of remedies each of which carries two numbers, for example:

Calc. 4/11
Lach. 4/12
Puls. 5/14
Sep. 5/11
Sul. 5/14

The interpretation is that *Calcarea* appeared in four of the rubrics under consideration, and achieved a total score of eleven, whilst *Sulphur* appeared in every rubric (which it usually does!) and achieved a total score of fourteen. This can be helpful in that one gets an idea of the relative intensity of each symptom under the remedies being considered.

Card Repertories

Attempts to mechanise and thereby speed up the repertorisation process were an inevitable development in homeopathy, and the first such attempt was the creation of a card repertory by William J. Guernsey in the late 1800's. This and the other card repertories that followed consisted of a large number of cards, each representing a rubric and bearing a series of punched-out holes in a particular configuration. When the rubrics in the case had been chosen, the relevent cards would be picked out of the box and placed one behind the other. Where the light was seen to shine through any of the holes, this meant that the remedy which that hole represented was to be found in every rubric chosen.

Considering the amount of labour that went into producing the various card repertories they have been pitifully neglected and now look set to become totally obsolete with the advent of computerisation. Probably the best-known and certainly the most comprehensive card repertory, based on Kent's, was created and developed by Dr. Jugal Kishore of Delhi. This repertory, which is still available, contains about 10,000 cards and even manages to represent the different grades of type as they are found in the book version.

Computerisation

The process of repertorisation is totally mechanical, which is why there now exist computer programmes to replace the books. However, the real skill of repertory work lies in the *selection of the symptoms and their interpretation into rubrics,* which requires a good working knowledge of the repertory being used as well as an accurate perception of what has to be cured in the patient.

The main advantage of computer repertories is still, therefore, a matter of speed - a case may be analysed at least three different ways on a computer in far less than the time it would take to do a single comprehensive repertorisation manually. This allows for totality repertorisations to be carried out far more frequently than would otherwise be possible, as it makes little difference to a computer whether the rubric being repertorised contain twenty remedies or two hundred.

Further levels of sophistication have been introduced in recent years which permit homeopaths to carry out analyses using computer software that would be impossible using the book versions. For instance, it is possible to determine which groups and families of remedies feature strongly in a case (see *Group Analysis* and *Thematic Prescribing*) and to change the relative weighting given to certain categories of materia medica so that the smaller remedies are not always obscured by the mighty polychrests.

Of the various software programmes now available, the *MacRepertory* system produced in the U.S.A. and the *C.A.R.A.* system produced in England are two of the most widely used. They share many features in common, including the ability to choose from a large range of different repertory authors and an increasingly vast database of materia medica information, making it possible to switch from repertory to materia medica and back again in the space of a few seconds.

The *RADAR* programme is another popular piece of repertory software which contains an 'expert system' designed to mimic the case analysis strategies of George Vithoulkas.

Disadvantages of Repertorisation
There are several drawbacks to repertorisation, the first one being that it can be extremely time consuming when carried out manually. The second is that in order to fit them into the format of a repertory, many symptoms have had to be broken down into their component parts. This means that the prescriber is often unaware of the context in which the symptom originally appeared in the provings. Knerr's *Repertory* to Hering's *Guiding Symptoms* contains a larger number of symptoms in their complete form than most other repertories, but because of this it is even more cumbersome to use.

A third drawback is that in order to use a repertory successfully it is necessary to interpret symptoms into rubrics accurately, bearing in mind that the compiler has already carried out a similar process of translation when creating the repertory. The difficulty is that in many instances we cannot be certain exactly what Kent, for example, had in mind when he coined the rubrics 'illusions of fancy' or 'wearisome' or 'repulsive mood'.

Further Reading

Bidwell
How to Use the Repertory
Jain Publishing Co., New Delhi, India

Castro
Encyclopaedia of Repertories
Jain Publishing Co., New Delhi, India

P. Coats
The Homeopathic Aide-Memoire
C.W. Daniel Co. Ltd., Saffron Walden, Essex

B.D. Desai
How to Find The Similimum with Boger-Boenninghausen's Repertory
B. Jain Publishers, New Delhi, India

Sequential Prescribing

You take exception to the number of remedies used in my last case, and want to know "which cured the case"? Will you get a long ladder and put it up against the side of your house, and mount it so as to get into your house by the top window; and when you have safely performed the feat, write and tell me which rung of that ladder enabled you to do it.

J. Compton-Burnett
Fifty Reasons for being a Homeopath

Definition
Under this heading I have included several related techniques which have the common aim of determining the sequence of events, traumas and circumstances that have contributed to a person's illness, and then systematically prescribing on each of these factors in a specific order.
See also: Layers

Introduction
Many cases present to homeopaths in which there appear to be a whole train of causative and contributory factors.that have collectively helped to shape that person's state of health, including emotional traumas, miasms, allopathic drugging, surgery, poor diet, and general toxicity. Certainly in some of these cases it is difficult to know even which methodology to apply, never mind what remedy to give! Practitioners past and present have developed various ways to navigate their way through these complicated cases, and below are some examples with which I am familiar.

James Compton-Burnett
Without doubt one of the master homeopaths of all time, James Compton-Burnett had to endure not only the ridicule of the allopaths, but the wrath of many within the homeopathic profession as well. His crime? To obtain spectacular cures in difficult cases by employing a series of different remedies, often given in fairly rapid succession. While he was not averse to alternating remedies now and again, for the most part he gave only one remedy at a time, according to the indications that he perceived in the case before him. His gift was simply that he perceived on many more levels than the vast majority of his colleagues, and was able to match those levels with different prescriptions.

Burnett, like Hahnemann before him, realised that symptom-matching was only one reason for prescribing a remedy, and there were many other reasons as well, all equally valid. He would, therefore, prescribe based on the miasms that he saw in the case, as well as the organ weaknesses, aetiologies and the type of pathology the patient had. He was remarkably flexible and seemingly unconcerned whether his patients needed just one remedy to get well or fifteen remedies, one after the other.

Burnett recorded many of his cases and was not ashamed to list all of the remedies he had given. In a typical chronic case, he would generally prescribe a course of one or more miasmatic remedies - usually the miasmatic nosode in a 30th potency or higher. This would be followed (or sometimes preceeded) by any aetiological remedies that the case might require - *Thuja* to deal with the vaccinal poison, for instance, *Bellis-perennis* if there was a history of injury, and so on.Now, having got the case moving in the direction of cure, he would seek to find any organ weaknesses that could benefit from a support remedy, usually in the form of a herbal tincture given in material doses. (The number of cases that he cured with these organ remedies alone are enough to fill several of his booklets.) In addition, he would study the particular pathology that the patient presented with, and look for a low-potency remedy or a series of remedies possessing an affinity with that type of disease process and the kind of tissue that was involved.

Probably the main reason why Burnett managed to upset just about everyone was his annoying habit of routinely curing cancerous tumours, epilepsy, tuberculosis, cataracts, varicose veins, alopecia and numerous other ailments, both chronic and acute, for which neither allopathy nor constitutional homeopathy alone had much to offer. The irony is that his method was not particularly radical - he simply utilised whatever approach seemed to fit the case at the time, changing direction as often as necessary to effect a cure.

Lisa Monck
More recently in England, Lisa Monck became frustrated in her efforts to cure chronic disease states using the single-remedy constitutional approach in which she had been trained. This led her to experiment with prescribing remedies in rapid succession according to the individual circumstances of the case, and she found she was able by this method to achieve far superior results in considerably less time.

Monck made many interesting observations on the process of healing, and she seemed to possess a different sense of what is possible than most of us. Once during a talk she described how she had learnt through her own experience to prescribe on what she saw, *when she saw it*. What this meant in practice was that she would often give a series of remedies and achieve an incredible amount of healing *during the actual consultation.*

She was of the opinion that when a person described a past trauma or some other factor important to their case, they would energetically be connected to that trauma or incident in that moment, and would be very receptive to an appropriate remedy. If, for example, someone described a past grief and she saw that some of that grief was still present, she might give *Ignatia* 10M on the spot. She would then wait a few minutes and see what came up next in the case. If the patient went on to mention a history of sexual abuse, and she saw that this was also still present energetically, she would give *Staphysagria* 10M there and then. In this way she might work through a whole series of remedies during the course of a one-hour consultation, and she felt that profound healing could take place in this way.

Pritam Singh

Another researcher in England who gave greater emphasis to prescribing on the miasmatic background, Pritam Singh developed his own sequential prescribing method which he attributed to his understanding of Hahnemann's *Chronic Diseases*. The 'Singh method', as it became known, has much in common with Burnett's approach, plus some other features besides, and it is described in detail in Roger Dyson and Jean Cole's book *Classical Homeopathy Revisited.*

The basic approach is to take note of the predominant miasms in the case, together with any other dyscrasias (taints) and to match them with indicated remedies, the reasoning being that until the miasms are addressed any other indicated remedies would be unlikely to fulfil their potential. Singh seemed to share Hahnemann's opinion that psora is the mother of all miasms, and even if another miasm was clearly active in the case he would generally treat the psoric aspect first, then follow up with other miasmatic nosodes as needed.

Having prescribed on the miasms, other dyscrasias are then addressed in order of importance to the case presenting. For example, if vaccination is considered to be a major factor then *Thuja* might be given to deal with this. *Radium-bromide* might be given to deal with radiation poisoning, *Folliculinum* for the effects of the contraceptive pill, and so on. One factor which Singh felt was very detrimental to health is the mercury amalgam used in dental fillings. He regarded this as a major contributory factor in many chronic cases, and prescribed *Hepar-sulph* in a range of potencies to counteract it.

The other key feature of the method is to support the miasmatic and dyscrasia prescribing with appropriate drainage remedies, with the intention of assisting elimination and strengthening organs such as the liver and kidneys where necessary.

Several things are striking when studying Singh's method. The first is that relatively few remedies are used, mostly major polychrests and nosodes with one or two exceptions. The idea is to get more action out of that limited range of remedies, rather than using an ever-increasing group of remedies as most homeopaths are tempted to do. The second is the use of descending potencies. This is something that Hahnemann experimented with, and Singh suggests that many unnecessary aggravations can be avoided by going down the potency scale. A typical prescription might be given in the 10M, 1M, and 200th potencies on one day, followed by 30, 12 and 6 on the next day.

Which leads to the next feature of this method - the frequent repetition of high potencies, and the rapidity with which one remedy follows another. It is normal practice in this approach to prescribe the chosen remedies *on consecutive days*. Typically, the patient might receive three or four remedies, including one or two nosodes, in a range of potencies during the first week, followed perhaps by a drainage remedy or a symptomatically-indicated remedy for a week, and then back to the nosodes again. Those used to giving a single dose of a single remedy and waiting a few months will find this aspect of Singh's approach somewhat alarming, but I have found that fears of provings and aggravations from this type of prescribing tend to be unfounded. It seems to me that the intention with which we give remedies has as much to do with their action as what we give.

Singh had an interesting idea that diseases arising in the first third of life were often due to environmental and nutritional factors, those commencing after age 30-35 were often inherited from the parents, and those arising after age 60-65 tended to be inherited from the grandparents or other distant relatives. He would attempt to match the depth of remedies he was prescribing to the level that he felt the disorder was arising from - i.e., the further back he was prescribing, the more he would look for a deeper-acting remedy. This is a novel hypothesis that, whilst it may not be literally true, provides a way of looking at cases that might prove useful.

Rudolph Verspoor

The Canadian homeopath Rudolph Verspoor has developed a system of sequential prescribing, inspired by the teachings of a Swiss practitioner, Dr. Jean Elmiger. The method evolved out of Elmiger's observation that chronic cases are often very difficult to cure by ordinary means due to the increased amount of allpathic drugging, vaccination and the stresses of modern life.

The emphasis of this approach is aetiological, and relies upon obtaining a chronological life-history of the patient, noting all of the significant traumas, be they mental, emotional or physical. Once the sequence of traumas has been established, the approach then is to prescribe on each of them in reverse order, using remedies that resonate with those aetiological factors. Verspoor feels that the sequence in which the remedies are prescribed is crucial, and that it is necessary to work backwards in time starting from the most recent trauma.

Several interesting observations have resulted from the work of these researchers, full details of which are to be found in Verspoor & Smith's book *Homeopathy Renewed: Cure and Prevention of Chronic Illness.* They found, for example, that in most cases when prescribing on the aetiologies the main remedy for each trauma will suffice - i.e., it is not necessary to individualise too much. If the trauma was a physical injury, *Arnica* would work most times, if it was a grief then *Ignatia* would suffice, etc. This tends to support my own experience that when the aetiology in a case is clear and direct, it can over-ride sympotomatology as a reason for prescribing.

Another observation they found, which again I would tend to concur with, is that unresolved *emotional* shocks are the most frequent causes of chronic illness, and when these are systematically and effectively treated with corresponding remedies, the greatest improvements in health tend to follow. Verspoor also states that the higher the potency, the greater the ability the remedy has to go back in time, which is an interesting idea but not one that I have been able to prove one way or the other.

The prescribing technique involves giving each aetiological remedy in a range of potencies, usually ascending the potency scale as in 30-200-1M-10M, each potency being given on successive days. A month or so interval is allowed to elapse before the next remedy is given in a similar fashion. If miasms are felt to be a factor in the case, these will be treated at some stage with the corresponding nosodes. Elmiger had a theory that the nosodes worked best if given during particular seasons corresponding to the miasms - *Psorinum* in the autumn, *Tuberculinum* in winter, *Medorrhinum* in spring and *Syphilinum* during summer. No mention is made of *Carcinosin*, which is probably my most frequently-prescribed nosode these days.

Conclusion

I have experimented with variations on all of the the methods described above, and my experience suggests that they are all valid approaches that can sometimes work wonders in cases where a single remedy approach seems to achieve very little. Many homeopaths will look back over their chronic cases and find that they have, in fact, been prescribing 'sequentially' without really being aware of it, moving from one approach to another to meet the demands of a particular case. I include these ideas here in order to stimulate further research and to encourage the reader to explore the boundaries of what might be possible in the future. Homeopathy is, after all, still in its infancy as a therapeutic system.

Further Reading

Dr. H.L. Chitkara
Best of Burnett - A Compilation of Burnett's Writings
B. Jain Publishers Ltd, New Delhi, India

R. Verspoor & P.L. Smith
Homeopathy Renewed: Cure and Prevention of Chronic Illness
Norsona Academy, Ontario, Canada

R. Dyson & J. Cole
Classical Homeopathy Revisited
Winter Press, London

J. Stallick
A.I.D.S. - The Homeopathic Challenge
Ribble Press, England

Specifics

Definition
'Near-specifics' is probably a more accurate name for this method. A remedy is prescribed on the basis that it nearly always works when given in similar circumstances, the assumption being that those circumstances produce a reasonably predictable remedy-image in the majority of cases, e.g. *Arnica* in physical injury.

Prescribing Technique
This is variable. Specifics are virtually always indicated in therapeutic or first-aid situations, and their range of effectiveness doesn't seem to extend further than this. When used within their limitations, specifics are ideal for over the counter prescribing, in that they generally come ready-packaged with a recommended potency and dosage, and may be instantly prescribed by anyone.

When to use Specifics
Specifics seem to be most appropriately used under the following circumstances:

1) In first-aid situations.
2) In a therapeutics situation (i.e. when the disease is to be treated rather than the patient) where there are no clear indications for another remedy.
3) When it is impossible to take a full case for some reason, and you wish to 'tide the patient over' with something rather than doing nothing.
4) In high-turnover prescribing situations where there is insufficient time for proper individualisation (general practitioners and pharmacists will find they can incorporate a fair amount of homeopathy into their existing practices by learning how to use specifics and therapeutics).

Examples of Specifics
Some of the specifics I would not wish to be without:

Altitude sickness	*Coca* 12 p.r.n.
Backache of late pregnancy	*Bellis-perennis* 6 t.d.s.
Dislocations, tendency to	*Calc.-fluor.* 6x t.d.s.
Fever with sepsis	*Pyrogen* 200 p.r.n.
Glandular fever	*Carcin.* 200 t.d.s. x 2 days
Gout	*Urtica-urens* Ø 5 dps t.d.s.
Growing pains	*Calc-phos.* 6x t.d.s.

Gumboil	*Calc.-sulph* 6x 2h.
Haemorrhage, minor	*Ficus-religiosa* 1x p.r.n.
Ingrowing toenail	*Mag.-p.-aust.* 2M s.d.
Miscarriage, threatened	*Viburnum-op.* 200 p.r.n.
Nervous exhaustion	*Avena-sat.* Ø 5 dps t.d.s.
Nosebleed	*Melilotus* 200 p.r.n.
Phlebitis, simple acute	*Hamam.* 30 (Ø ext.) p.r.n.
Prostate enlargement	*Sabal-serrulata* 3x t.d.s.
Ringworm	*Bacillinum* 200 c.s.d.
Scar tissue problems	*Thiosiaminum* 6x t.d.s.
Toothache	*Plantago* 3x p.r.n.
Warts all over hands	*Ferrum-picricum* 6 t.d.s.
Wrist ganglion	*Ruta* 50M s.d.

General Notes

It is worth mentioning that, bizzare as it may seem, specifics are not always transferrable from one practitioner to another. I have often been told of a specific which works "every time" for some practitioner, only to find it fail miserably in my own practice, and I have occasionally received similar feedback from others who have tried out my specifics and been disappointed. I cannot explain this phemomenon, and would welcome contributions from anyone who can.

Individualisation plays such an important role in successful prescribing that some homeopaths have denied that such a thing as specifics can be legitimately employed in homeopathy. My experience thus far suggests they have a valid place, so I include the method here and will let you, the reader, decide for yourself.

Further Reading

R. B. Bishamber Das
Select Your Remedy
Vishwamber Free Home Dispensary, New Delhi, India

M. Fayazuddin
Diseased Conditions as we meet in Everyday Practice
B. Jain Publishers Ltd, New Delhi

J. N. Shinghal
Quick Bed-Side Prescriber
B. Jain Publishers Ltd, New Delhi

S. Siddhantalankar
First-Aid Specifics of Homeopathic & Biochemic Treatment
Vijay Krishna Lakhanpal, 4/24 Asafali Rd, New Delhi

I. Watson
A Remedy for Everything!
A Remedy for Everything Else!
Recorded Seminars, available in Audiotape and CD formats
www.ianwatsonseminars.com

Symptom Similarity

The Totality of Symptoms insisted on by Hahnemann as the basis of correspondence does not refer only to their numerical sum, but to their relative importance

John H. Clarke
Dictionary of Practical Materia Medica

Definition
This method involves prescribing a remedy because the symptoms of the patient bear similarity to symptoms found within the remedy-picture.

Introduction
I still sometimes catch myself, when talking to people about homeopathy, blatantly stating that there is little more to it than matching symptoms produced in a proving to the symptoms encountered in a diseased individual. If only it were that simple! Computers would already be capable of replacing prescribers if homeopathy were as straightforward as that.

The symptoms in the case commonly form the primary basis for the prescription, but very often they do not, as the chapters on ætiologies and miasms, for instance, will show. To me, symptom-similarity is just one variation on the theme of similars, and there are many others. Not only that, there are many different ways in which symptoms can be manipulated to locate the curative remedy.

Totality of Symptoms
The 'totality of symptoms' is one of the most misleading concepts in homeopathy, for it suggests that if all the symptoms of a case are gathered together and a remedy is found that contains a similar gathering, that remedy will be the curative similimum. Hahnemann wrote "..........so that each individual case of disease is most surely, radically, rapidly and permanently annihilated and removed only by a medicine capable of producing (in the human system) in the most similar and complete manner the totality of its symptoms, which at the same time are stronger than the disease." (*Organon of Medicine*, paragraph 27)

Up to a point this is true, but it is also a rather cumbersome procedure given that a chronically sick patient may present page after page of symptoms.

Provided they are all accurately recorded and their equivalent is painstakingly located in the materia medica, a curative prescription can be found in this way. It soon becomes obvious, however, that this method is as inefficient as it is time-consuming, hence various ways of streamlining the process have been worked out which render it less labour-intensive yet more consistently effective.

Hahnemann obviously discovered this for himself, as he writes[1] in *The Organon*, paragraph 104: "When the totality of the symptoms *that specially mark and distinguish the case of disease* or, in other words, when the picture of the disease, whatever be its kind, is once accurately sketched, the most difficult part of the task is accomplished. The physician has then the picture of the disease, especially if it be a chronic one, always before him to guide him in his treatment; he can investigate it in all its parts *and can pick out the characteristic symptoms*, in order to oppose *to these* .... a homeopathically chosen medicinal substance." (my italics).

In other words, the totality of symptoms (i.e. all of them) must be taken down, but only in order that a portion of those symptoms may then be selected and utilised for finding the similimum. Virtually every homeopath I know does exactly this, yet I still hear and read of the totality of symptoms as being the basis of a prescription. If the truth be told, a *selected partiality* of the given totality of symptoms provides a more reliable guide to the curative remedy than the totality itself. That being the case, how then are we to decide which symptoms to select and which to ignore? What constitutes a "characteristic symptom"? This is truly one of the grey areas of homeopathy, and one which many prescribers have attempted to clarify.

Characteristic Symptoms

My dictionary defines as *characteristic* "that (which) serves to indicate character; distinctive; typical; a distinguishing peculiarity or quality." Characteristic symptoms seem to have to do with uniqueness, individuality and sometimes rarity or peculiarity. Selecting the characteristics of a given case involves paying attention to that which makes the case unique, or unusual, unexpected or particularly striking. Hahnemann gives his own clues as to which symptoms should be chosen, referring[2] to "the *more striking, singular, uncommon and peculiar* (characteristic) signs and symptoms ...."

It might be that a certain symptom is so clear and *striking* that it begs your attention, or it might be *uncommon* in the context of the type of illness or the type of patient being treated. Occasionally a symptom that is physiologically inexplicable will prove to be the key to the case. The main idea to keep in mind is that certain things are common to virtually everyone, and other things are unique to the individual.

A famous analogy tells of the fact that all human beings have in common two eyes, two ears, a nose, a mouth, lips, teeth, hair etc. All of these can be said to be "common" to human beings, and equivalent to "common" symptoms such as are found in many patients - headache, lethargy, insomnia, chilliness, constipation etc. In addition to these, there also exists in everyone some "distinguishing peculiarities or qualities" which enable us to recognise that individual and differentiate him/her from everyone else. It might be that the teeth are crooked, or that the breath smells peculiar, the voice is husky, the eyes look in different directions or the lips are full and voluptuous. Everyone has certain features which, when they appear together in a certain configuration, permit immediate recognition of the individual. If a similar approach is taken to the symptoms in a case, the characteristics will be found.

One of the problems in homeopathy is that the art of individualisation and recognising characteristic symptoms is very difficult to teach to someone else - often the best that anyone can do is to draw a student's attention to the necessity for it, then leave them to discover it for themselves by direct experience. The situation is similar to my walking into a field of fifty sheep and attempting to identify each of them as individuals. The problem I have is that they all look alike to me! In other words, all that I notice are the signs which are "common" to sheep - the wool, the tendency to run away, the placid expression etc. However, an observant farmer would quite easily be able to pick out single members of the flock, pointing out certain features that *obviously* (to him) make each one an individual. Thus speaks the voice of experience.

Keynote Symptoms
I have never been quite sure whether keynotes and characteristics are one and the same thing or whether the originators of the terms had something different in mind for each. The word keynote is actually a musical term referring to the 'first (i.e. lowest) note of the scale of any key, which forms the basis of, and gives its name to, the key itself'. My understanding of 'keynote prescribing', is that a prescription is based on one or a few outstanding (i.e. characteristic) symptoms of the case which are known to be strongly indicative of a particular remedy, especially when only one or a few remedies are known to have that symptom or group of symptoms.

Keynote prescribing has had an unjustifiably bad press in the homeopathic literature, most notably from Kent, and it seems to have become something of a lost art in recent years. The great masters of keynote prescribing were the likes of Lippe, Allen, Guernsey and Nash, to name but a few.

Origins of Keynotes

Keynotes are created from three main sources:

1) Provings:- i.e. those symptoms which appeared in a wide cross-section of provers taking the same remedy. An example would be the heat and redness of *Belladonna,* a symptom which affected a great many of the provers in various different locations.

2) Verified Symptoms:- i.e. those symptoms which may have appeared in many or in just a few provers, but which have been successfully *cured* by that remedy in practice on many occasions. An example would be the "painful cracks in the right-hand corner of the mouth" which Burnett produced in himself when proving *Cundurango,* and which led him to prescribe the remedy successfully in numerous cases of cancer where a similar symptom was present.

3) Clinical Indications:- those symptoms or conditions which *never* appeared in the provings, but which have been repeatedly cured by the remedy in practice when it was prescribed on other symptoms present. Virtually all of the ætiological indications were discovered in this way, some of which have become guiding symptoms to the remedy. Examples would be "ailments following smallpox vaccination" indicating *Thuja,* "mental changes following head injury" indicating *Natrum sulph,* and "ill effects of puncture wounds" indicating Ledum. The latter I believe was first observed by Teste, and has since proved to be one of the most reliable and invaluable indications for the remedy.

Leading Keynotes

Many times I have prescribed a remedy successfully on a few keynote symptoms alone. Keynotes also provide invaluable differentiation between several remedies which appear to be well-indicated on other grounds.

Most remedies have one or two symptoms which are so well-verified that they suggest the use of that remedy almost regardless of the rest of the case, when outstanding in the patient. The literature is scattered with examples of cured cases where the prescription was based on just one such symptom. Nearly always when a symptom such as this is present, the rest of the case will be found to correspond to the remedy for which the symptom is a keynote.

Examples of leading keynotes:

Symptoms alternate sides	*Lac-caninum*
Symptoms worse for motion	*Bryonia*
Pain under right scapula	*Chelidonium*
Pulse out of proportion to temperature	*Pyrogen*
Nausea with clean tongue	*Ipecacuanha*
Abdomen feels drawn by a string to spine	*Plumbum*
Symptoms worse between 2am and 4am	*Kali-carbonicum*
Triangular red tip on tongue	*Rhus-tox*
Feels unusually well before an attack	*Psorinum*

Case Examples

Recently I treated a woman with almost constant, severe nausea during pregnancy, worse from the smell of cooking food and with a hollow empty feeling in the stomach. It seemed like a clear case of *Sepia*, so I gave it and nothing happened. Looking at the miasmatic background together with the hollow feeling and the *persistent* nausea I gave *Psorinum*. Again nothing happened. I questioned her again about each symptom in turn, finally asking "what, apart from the nausea, is the most outstanding symptom you have?" She pondered this and replied "well, the strange thing is that *so long as I keep eating* I feel O.K." On this I prescribed *Anacardium* 10M and she was fine within a couple of days.

I was once compelled to prescribe *Thuja* to a man with prostate trouble who volunteered the fact that his urine came out *in a forked stream*, and it helped him enormously. I was led to *Thuja* in another case where the symptom *weeps on hearing music* was very marked, and it produced a curative response even though it appeared to cover very few of the other symptoms present.

Strange, Rare and Peculiar Symptoms

Symptoms only become strange or rare or peculiar in the context of the individual in whom they are found. For example, singing in the street would be strange in a bank manager but fairly common in a drunkard. Provided the prescriber is familiar with the signs and symptoms common to disease, peculiar symptoms are fairly easy to locate, particularly in acute illnesses. Thirstlessness during fever is the classic example; a migraine headache *relieved* by noise or light would be another. In chronic disease, the strange symptoms often go undetected or unnoticed because of the numberless ways in which individuals present with a similar disorder. Here the emphasis is not so much on "what is strange in this illness?" but rather "what is strange in this individual?"

Case Examples

My former wife, Sally, brought home the case she had taken of a forty-seven year old man who complained of "bad kidneys" and an undiagnosed respiratory problem, both of many years standing. He had swelling and tenderness in the kidney region and a history of acute nephritis. His urine tended to be cloudy. Frequent urging at night. Prone to constipation; occasional knife-like pains up the rectum, worse at night. He had a feeling of pressure on the chest and a weak, sick feeling in the chest area. Obstructed nose with thick, white mucus. Feet tingled in bed. He sweated a lot, worse after a warm drink; sometimes he sweated so much he had to dry himself with a towel. Occasionally he would pass stools mixed with a little blood and mucus. History of pneumonia, boils and warts in childhood.

There seemed to be two outstanding "characteristic" symptoms in this case, one of which was undoubtedly "strange, rare and peculiar". That was what he described as a "weak, sick feeling in the chest", which he had only mentioned in passing but which Sally had diligently recorded verbatim. Sickness in the stomach is common enough, but *in the chest?* This had to be the key to the case. Kent's repertory revealed eighteen remedies having this symptom (p. 506), all in low type except for *Crocus, Mercurius* and *Rhus tox,* which appeared in italics.

The second characteristic earned its place owing to the incredible *intensity* of the symptom - he sweated so profusely he had to dry himself off with a towel! How can you ignore a symptom like that? Those two combined led us quickly to *Mercurius,* which covered the other outstanding symptoms clearly and was prescribed in the 200th and later the 1M potencies with wonderful improvement in every respect.

Cases like this teach you that it always pays to reflect on a case, to look at it from several different angles *before* you start ploughing through the repertory or materia medica. Training yourself to do this saves much unnecessary work in the long run. If a case has been well-taken you have all the information needed to make a good prescription, but the art of prescribing on symptoms lies in sifting the wheat from the chaff.

Sally once treated an elderly lady who had awful difficulty walking due to the fact that her toes would bend involuntarily as soon as she put her foot to the ground. Remedies prescribed on her general state produced little improvement, so we determined to track down that strange symptom. After a lengthy search we found something akin to it listed under *Badiaga.* The only thing I knew about *Badiaga* was that it had a cough with expectoration that literally flies out of the mouth, which she didn't have. We gave it to her regardless and she showed a marked improvement.

I am often surprised how frequently patients will divulge a 'strange, rare or peculiar' symptom without either patient or practitioner being aware of it. I treated a woman for several months with limited success, who had a multitude of physical and emotional symptoms. After retaking the case yet again and learning nothing knew, I decided to comb through the casenotes from all the previous visits and see what I had missed. The thing that struck me straight away was a phrase she had used time and time again, and which I had always written down but paid little attention to in the analysis. What she had said was, in describing her energy state, "I feel half dead". Suddenly it resonated with something I had read somewhere, and sure enough, there it was in the Mind section of Kent's Repertory: 'Delusions, body alive on one side, buried on the other'. The remedy was *Stramonium*, and she responded to it wonderfully.

Complete Symptoms

Boenninghausen applied his lawyer's brain to the problem of finding the homeopathic similimum, and he left us several useful tools to enhance the process. One of these I shall refer to as "CLAMS", the interpretation of which is given below:

Concomitant
Location
Aetiology
Modality
Sensation

Boenninghausen had the idea that every symptom is a manifestation of the disorder in the whole person, and if each symptom is coming from the same source then each could theoretically be used to lead back to that source. Just as the spokes of a wheel appear to be separate and far apart at their outer aspect, all are joined as one in the centre. For practical purposes, he recommended that during casetaking every symptom be completed as fully as possible in each of the above aspects.

Usually the patient will offer one or two aspects spontaneously - "I have a splitting *(sensation)* headache *(location)*". What you need to complete the picture is one or more modalities and perhaps an aetiology or concomitant. It is rare to complete a symptom in all five aspects, but I always aim for three as a minimum. There is definitely truth in the statement that a case well taken is more than half cured.

I find 'CLAMS' an extremely useful tool to help me ensure I have as complete a picture as it is possible to obtain. For a while I had it written on my telephone pad so that when taking acute cases over the phone I would be reminded to fill in the blank areas before hanging up. After practising this for a while it becomes second nature, and my brain now tends to know automatically when I have a complete symptom and when something is missing that I haven't enquired about.

Incidentally, a similar phenomenon seems to have pervaded my chronic casetaking as well. Quite often I have taken a case thoroughly but at the end of it I have had an uneasy feeling that there was something missing, not knowing what it could be. When this happens, I will now say to the patient something like: "I can't prescribe for you yet because there is something missing somewhere and I don't know what it is", and look at him or her expectantly. Invariably the patient will come up with something they hadn't thought to mention or had deliberately avoided, and the picture is completed. I've no idea how this works, but it's damn useful!

The Three-legged Stool

Hering introduced the idea of a three-legged stool into homeopathy. He suggested that *three* outstanding symptoms - keynotes, characteristics or whatever you like to call them - were all that was necessary in order to find a curative remedy. I always like to get a fourth symptom to clinch the case, but three seems to be a good minimum in most cases. Remember that three *common* symptoms are as good as useless - symptoms must always be weighed as well as counted!

Further Reading

H. C. Allen
Keynotes and Characteristics with Comparisons
Indian Books & Periodical Syndicate, New Delhi-110055, India

C. M. Boger
Boenninghausen's Characteristics and Repertory
Jain Publishing Co., New Delhi, India

A. Von Lippe
Keynotes of the Homeopathic Materia Medica
Jain Publishing Co., New Delhi, India

H. N. Guernsey
Keynotes to the Materia Medica
Jain Publishing Co., New Delhi-110055, India

E. B. Nash
Leaders in Homeopathic Therapeutics
Jain Publishing Co., New Delhi-110055, India

R. Gibson-Miller
Comparative Value of Symptoms in the Selection of the Remedy
Jain Publishing Co., New Delhi, India

P. Sankaran
Analysis and Evaluation of Symptoms
The Selection of the Simillimum and the Management of the Patient
Homeopathic Medical Publishers, Bombay, India

F. Vermeulen
Concordant Materia Medica
Synoptic Materia Medica vols. 1 & 2
Merlijn Publishers, Netherlands

Tautopathy

Definition

Tauto = 'the same'

This method is really a variation of isopathy, the difference being that tautopathy refers specifically to the prescription of a potentised *drug or toxin* that a person has ingested at some time previously.

When to Use Tautopathy

There are several situations in which tautopathy may be usefully employed, generally as an adjunct to rather than a replacement for other forms of homeopathic treatment.

My starting point with any patient, whatever drugs or vaccines they have taken, is always that if you see a *clearly* indicated remedy, then give it. My belief is that if the organism is able to put out a clear, single remedy image in spite of drugs and so on, that is a good sign and they will very likely respond well to the remedy. It is not necessary to 'antidote' everything the person has ever taken in the way of medication - the vast majority of it will have left no long-term effects once it has been discontinued. My colleague and friend Robert Davidson taught me a golden rule that is always worth remembering in this context: *if it ain't broke, don't fix it!*

Aetiological Prescription

If a patient reports that they have 'never been well since' taking a certain drug, inhaling some kind of fumes, receiving a vaccination or swallowing a poisonous chemical, all of these are direct ætiologies and the treatment should include the causation as far as possible. It has been found by clinical experience that the ill-effects of many drugs, toxins and treatments can be antidoted by a remedy based on the symptoms of the patient. For example, *Pulsatilla* is known to be a leading remedy for patients who have suffered from taking iron, *Nux vomica* for the abuse of narcotics and laxatives, and *Thuja* for the effects of smallpox vaccination.

The following case illustrates the point that a remedy prescribed on the symptom-picture will take care of the ill-effects of drugs, provided it is clearly indicated.

A four year old boy had been feverish, sweating, grumpy and off his food for several days. He had an increased thirst and was restless and very unhappy with himself. All the symptoms had come on shortly after his receiving cholera and typhoid vaccines, and the family were due to go abroad in two days. The most striking thing of all was that he wrapped himself around his mother like a koala bear, and absolutely refused to be examined. I looked in the rubric 'Aversion to being looked at' in Kent's *Repertory* and *Antimonium tartaricum* caught my attention, my having read something in a booklet a few weeks earlier about its use following vaccination. In Phatak's *Materia Medica* under *Ant. tart.* is the indication 'after vaccination when *Thuja* fails and *Silica* is not indicated', and also the symptom 'clings to attendants'. A single dose of *Ant. tart.* 200 was given and he was fine within twelve hours. I have since used *Antimonium tart.* in several cases of 'ailments following vaccination' with equal success, and have added it to the rubric in my repertory in italics.

I think it is vital that we always record our results in cases like this, and I hope that a mechanism will soon be created whereby every practitioner's clinical observations can be pooled, to the enormous benefit of everyone. The arrival of computer technology means that information such as this could be stored and accessed in a way previously never dreamed of, yet at the moment we are far less diligent in recording and sharing our experiences with one another than were the practitioners of the past.

One of the major problems which homeopaths face today is in dealing with the ill-effects of literally hundreds of new chemicals, drugs, vaccines, anæsthetics and so on. It is not at all uncommon for a patient who is chronically sick to be taking several drugs simultaneously, many of which have been prescribed to overcome the effects of their predecessors. Incredibly, traditional homeopathic methods can often overcome the effects of drugs and restore the patient to health, but tautopathy is a technique which can be extremely useful in cases where a clearly indicated remedy cannot be found or where remedies fail to act satisfactorily.

The most dramatic results are achieved with tautopathy in cases where the drug or toxin was the direct ætiology for the patient's complaint. As long as the nature of the substance is known, it can be potentised and given back to the patient like any other remedy.

Case Examples
A woman in her sixties came to see me and told me her "gullet had shrunk". When she tried to swallow, food became lodged behind the sternum, causing a "hot" pain which went through to the back. The pain was relieved by regurgitating the food. On drinking she often had spasmodic attacks of

hiccoughs. She had frequent eructations of wind; a sensation of a lump in the throat, not relieved by swallowing; easy satiety and a tendency towards constipation.

About eight years previously she had an internal investigation of the gullet which caused lacerations and punctured her right lung. The lung collapsed and she developed pleurisy as a result. This had left her with a tendency to get out of breath easily, and soreness in the chest on deep inspiration. While I was studying the case I gave *Arnica* 200 followed by *Calendula* 30 on the basis of the past trauma, and this relieved the soreness in the chest but produced no other change. On repertorising the symptoms *Natrum muriaticum* seemed best indicated but it was given with no result. *Kali carbonicum* and *Lachesis* were also tried but without relief.

I decided to question her for further information about the onset of the trouble. It transpired that approximately one year after the lung episode she had "an attack of arthritis" in the right hip. She was given Naprosyn (a non-steroid anti-inflammatory drug). As soon as she started taking it she developed an awful burning in the oesophagus. After a week the drug was stopped, but ever since then she had had the difficulty swallowing, pain behind the sternum and feeling of a lump in the throat. In fact, she assured me she had "never been well since".

On hearing this I obtained a bottle of *Naprosyn* 30 and sent her three doses to take over a 24-hour period. The next day her husband called to ask "what the hell have you given to my wife?" He said she had never looked so ill since the Asian 'flu thirty years ago! I tried to sound confident that all would be well, and said to wait another day. The next day the woman rang me and proudly declared she had just eaten toast without any problem for the first time in years. She had no further trouble at all for about three months - she could swallow anything, there was no pain or regurgitation, her wind disappeared and her general health improved considerably. Then she had a partial relapse after the sudden death of a close friend, which *Ignatia* 200 took care of very quickly. I sent further *Naprosyn* 30 to hold, but she never needed to take it.

This case demonstrates the typical result with a tautopathic presription in a 'never been well since' situation, i.e. marked initial aggravation followed by rapid and dramatic improvement.

Another patient of mine suffered a severe attack of vomiting and diarrhoea immediately after coating her garden fence with kreosote. Her symptoms were so severe that I was tempted to prescribe *Veratrum album* which covered the prostration and violent evacuations fairly well. However, on reading Clarke's *Materia Medica* I found similar symptoms listed under *Kreosotum*, so I gave her a few doses of *Kreosotum* 30 instead. The result was that she ceased vomiting immediately and gradually recovered over the next few days. About two weeks later she had no return of the acute symptoms but said that she still didn't feel quite right since the poisoning, so I gave her a dose of *Kreosotum* 10M which picked her up completely.

Ill-Effects of Vaccines
The vaccines which are currently in use are all polychrest remedies, in as much as they have all caused and are therefore capable of curing a multitude of acute and chronic health problems. I have used potentised *B.C.G.* (anti-tubercular) vaccine in numerous cases with good results. A fairly common ill effect of this vaccine is the onset of symptoms resembling rheumatoid arthritis, with usually several joints being affected and wandering pains. I have seen this condition totally cured after a few doses of *B.C.G.* 30, where indicated remedies had failed to hold, and I have also seen juvenile acne respond well to *B.C.G.*. My colleague David Howell, who makes good use of tautopathy in his practice, treated an eleven year old girl whose growth had become completely stunted at the age of six. Tracing this back to the B.C.G. vaccine, he gave a single dose of *B.C.G.* 30, after which she grew two and a half inches in just three months.

The triple vaccine is just as ubiquitous in its effects on the organism, if not more so. Harris Coulter's book *D.P.T. - A shot in the Dark?* contains a catalogue of symptoms and diseases attributable to the vaccine, and makes distressing reading. I personally have treated chronic, recurring ear infections, recurring high fevers, chronic diarrhoea, allergic states, skin problems, chronic catarrh and 'glue ear' successfully with *D.P.T.* 30. Whenever I see a child whose troubles started around three or six months of age I am already thinking strongly of *D.P.T.* as a first prescription.

Remedy Reaction
It should be borne in mind that when a drug or toxin is a causative factor in the case, the patient will often be extremely sensitive to that same drug in potentised form, even years later. I once saw a patient who had reacted violently to the polio vaccine when it was administered, and it produced symptoms which were still present twenty-three years later! I gave him a dose of *Polio (Salk) Vaccine* 30 and he responded to it almost immediately. My experience in these cases has taught me that it is advisable to give tautopathic remedies in not too high potency to begin with, so as to minimise aggravations.

Intercurrent Remedy

Sometimes patients will present with a fairly clear remedy picture, but that remedy, on being prescribed, fails to act as well as it should or the patient soon relapses. This may suggest a miasmatic blockage in the case, but it could also be that a drug or other toxin that has been ingested in the past is preventing the remedy from acting fully. In cases like this, an intercurrent prescription of the drug in potency will clear the way and allow the indicated remedy to act as it should. I used this technique with a woman suffering from eczema who responded to the indicated constitutional remedy, *Calcarea Carbonica*, but relapsed very quickly. On the basis that she had been given penicillin on numerous occasions in the past, and knowing that it has a strong affinity for the skin, I prescribed *Penicillin* 200. To my surprise it actually produced a marked improvement in her condition, and when I gave *Calc. carb.* again subsequently, it completed the cure and there was no further relapse.

I have treated numerous patients with joint problems who at some time in the past have been given cortisone injections directly into the joints. Several of these patients have either failed to respond to treatment altogether, or have responded well generally but the joints which had been injected continued to be a problem. In these cases I have given a few doses of *Cortisone* 200 and it has either produced a marked improvement in the condition or has enabled further treatment to progress unhindered.

Some of our famous 'imponderabilia' can be usefully employed as intercurrent tautopathic prescriptions. For example, patients who have received multiple X-rays who fail to respond to treatment may well require a dose of potentised *X-ray;* cancer patients and others with a history of radiation exposure may require *Radium Bromide* and patients who have endured E.C.T. treatment in the past may prove difficult to treat until they have been given *Electricitas.*

Elimination of Toxins

It has been demonstrated[1] in experiments carried out in the 1950's and 60's that animals injected with sub-lethal doses of toxins such as arsenic or bismuth would eliminate far greater quantities of the poison in the urine or stools if they were then given the same substance in low potencies such as 4c, 5c and 7c. Whilst the investigation techniques are objectionable, the results suggest that tautopathy could prove effective in treating cases of poisoning, overdose and other forms of chemical toxicity.

It has been suggested by Drs. Tyler, Foubister and others that potencies of *Alumina* can be helpful to patients who have become poisoned with aluminium through the continued use of cooking utensils made from the metal. Given the extent to which we are now subjected to environmental toxins in one form or another, it would be worthwhile investigating the effectiveness of this technique on large samples of people.

Drug Withdrawal

There is plenty of empirical evidence that tautopathy will assist in the withdrawal of drugs and medications, particularly those that are generally difficult to withdraw such as tranquillizers or steroids. I have found that by giving the same drug in potentised form during the period of withdrawal the process can be hastened and made less traumatic for the patient than it might otherwise have been. My preferred technique is to give, say, *Prednisolone* 30 twice a week, whilst *gradually* reducing the dosage of the drug over a period of weeks or months as necessary. I have in some cases observed a reduction in the side-effects caused by a drug, even before the dosage was reduced, by giving it in potentised form in the above manner. These results tend to confirm that a tautopathic prescription can indeed enhance the elimination of a substance from the body. It would be a worthwhile project to test the effectiveness of this technique as a supportive measure in those withdrawing from other drugs such as heroin, for whom the withdrawal period is especially traumatic.

Further Reading

D. M. Foubister
Constitutional Effects of Anæsthesia
Indian Books & Periodicals Syndicate, New Delhi, India
The Significance of Past History in Homeopathic Prescribing
Homeopathic Medical Publishers, Bombay, India

R. Patel
What is Tautopathy?
Hahnemann Homeopathic Pharmacy, India

Thematic Prescribing

The homeopaths of the future will not be 'unprejudiced observers'. They will be self-aware participants in the magical interaction that occurs between practitioner, client and remedy. Furthermore, they will no longer rely only on that which can be perceived 'objectively' with the senses. They will learn to fine-tune their inner faculties, and practice with confidence and accuracy based on their understanding and awareness of energy.

Ian Watson

Definition
This method encompasses a number of different ways of grouping remedies together according to certain themes or patterns, and matching these to corresponding themes and patterns found in patients.
See also: Group Analysis

Introduction
In recent years there has been a considerable expansion of the materia medica, and whilst the repertories have struggled to keep pace with all the new remedies being introduced, the prescriber's job is not made any easier by the introduction of literally hundreds of unfamiliar remedy pictures every year. One way in which homeopaths have found that they can integrate a large amount of information into practice is to learn remedies in groups and families of different kinds, rather than attempting to learn every remedy individually. This is not a new idea by any means - Farrington's *Clinical Materia Medica,* for example, discusses remedies that fall into natural groups such as snake venoms and remedies from related plant species. Cooper and Burnett also studied remedies in this way, recognising that several plants from the same family were liable to have certain symptoms and affinities in common.

These hints from some of the old masters have inspired contemporary homeopaths to develop these themes even further, and to extend them beyond being simply aids to learning, into the realms of case analysis and actual prescribing in fairly sophisticated ways. The basic idea is to categorise remedies according to some particular theme, and then to look for a similar theme in a patient. Once the theme itself is identified, the job of finding the most similar remedy is made a lot easier because *only the remedies related to that theme* need be considered. As an example, it has become commonplace for homeopaths to say "this person needs a spider remedy" or "that person needs a mineral". Having matched the person to a specific *group* of remedies, the task then is to use the symptoms of the case to differentiate *within that group.*

The groups and themes that have been developed are many and varied, and reflect the interests of different prescribers. I will mention only a few of the better-known themes with which I have some personal experience.

The Circle

The circle is a system of analysis based on the traditional four elements - earth, air, fire and water. The Israeli homeopath Joseph Reeves is credited with associating homeopathic remedies with these themes initially, and in recent years this work has been developed and extended in the U.K. by Jeremy Scherr, David Mundy, Misha Norland and others.

The four elements are understood to be inter-related and complementary, and they represent the four basic ways in which energy-as-matter manifests. They are sometimes referred to as the four qualities - dry, cold, hot and damp. (It is interesting to note that they overlap considerably with the ancient Chinese five-element system, where the types are described as earth, water, metal, wood and fire.) Once the nature of these basic qualities have been understood, it is then possible to describe remedies and patients in terms of the relative emphasis of the four elements. Remedies can be grouped by noting, for example, which element is dominant or lacking. *Natrum-mur.,* by this method, would have a predominance of water, whilst *Belladonna,* with all its heat, redness and fevers, would clearly be in the fiery group.

Case analysis based on the circle attempts to gain an understanding of the balance of these energetic qualities in the patient, and then to find a remedy or group of remedies with a corresponding balance. The circle has been extended to include many correspondences of organs, systems, diseases, temperaments etc., and someone who is well versed in it has a considerable advantage over a homeopath who only sees symptoms as symptoms. What the circle, and some of the other ways of grouping remedies provide, is a framework for understanding the energetic imbalance within a patient which, to my mind, is an essential skill for a practitioner of what is, after all, an energy medicine.

Planetary Diagnosis

This technique has been developed and refined by Robin Murphy, and instead of being based on four basic types, it is based on seven. These are represented by the seven planets of the ancients, corresponding to the seven days of the week. These are the sun (sunday), moon (monday), mars (tuesday), mercury (wednesday), jupiter (thursday), venus (friday) and saturn (saturday). One of the most interesting aspects of this system is that it allows for the diagnosis of both 'fixed' planets that are determined by the day and time of a person's birth, and also transitory planets that are passing influences. This enables the prescriber to diagnose inherent organ weaknesses and other susceptibilities with a fair degree of accuracy, and also to differentiate between diseases that are a result of constitutional tendencies from those that are acquired due to other causes.

As with the elements of the circle, each of the seven planets represents a particular type or quality of energy, and has a wide range of correspondences associated with it. The moon, for example, is considered to rule the brain, stomach, and breasts; the menstrual cycle, conception and fertility; sleep, dreams and the unconcious realm; and disorders such as addictions, insomnia, haemorrhage and travel sickness. Each planet also has a corresponding metal and gemstone, and a range of herbal and homeopathic remedies that will tend to resonate with that particular type of energy. Another intriguing aspect of planetary diagnosis is that associations can be made with times of the day, days of the week and specific stages of life, which can help to illuminate many of the otherwise inexplicable modalities that exist in our materia medica.

Case examples
I once treated someone with an undiagnosed neuro-muscular problem, with varying degrees of weakness in the limbs and transient pains. After trying several remedies based on the symptom-picture to no avail, I studied the planets that corresponded to the patient's date and time of birth, which turned out to be mercury in both cases. On this basis, and knowing that mercury has an affinity with the nervous system, I gave the corresponding planetary metal, in the form of *Mercurius-vivus* 6c, and it produced a marked and lasting improvement in her condition.

My colleague Anne Waters tried a similar approach in a case of chronic rheumatoid arthritis which indicated remedies failed to alleviate. The patient was born on a Saturday, which suggests she would have a constitutional tendency to problems corresponding to the energy of the planet saturn. These include problems with the bones and skeletal system, and a tendency to stiffness and degeneration of tissue. Anne prescribed the planetary metal of saturn, which is lead, in the form of *Plumbum-metallicum* and *Plumbum-iodatum*, combined together in the 6th potency. The patient reported that this remedy gave a huge amount of relief, and was decidedly more effective than the other remedies she had taken. Cases like this one serve to illustrate how the potential curative properties of metals and other substances are not always confined to the symptomatic indications brought out in provings.

In another case I treated someone with a chronic tickly cough which the usual cough remedies failed to cure. Tracing it back to its origin, the cough had begun on a Saturday, and on this basis I gave *Ceanothus* 6c which produced a curative result. The remedy was chosen because in the planetary system the main organ associated with saturn is the spleen, and this reminded me of a number cases that Burnett describes in his writings where the patient had what he termed a 'splenic cough'.

Chakra Diagnosis
Another map of seven which many homeopaths have found helpful describes the seven chakras, or energy-centres, and this system provides another way of grouping a large number of phenomena and their corresponding remedies into a manageable number of basic themes.

The chakras are considered to be places within the human energy system where life energy is concentrated and filtered, and they are a kind of interface between a person's psychological state and their physical body. Each chakra has an associated endocrine gland and other related organs, as well as a correspondence with a particular type of emotional energy. When, for example, the emotion becomes suppressed, the energy flow at that centre will be impeded, and there will be a corresponding effect on the related endocrine gland and other organs.

Although the chakras were described thousands of years ago in the ancient vedic texts, fields such as psycho-neuro-immunology have only recently begun to confirm how truly inseparable the mind and body are. Homeopaths, of course, have long recognised this inter-relationship, but familiarity with the chakras enables a far greater depth of understanding in this area. I have come to believe that the anatomy and physiology of the energy system, of which the chakras are an important aspect, ought to be a standard part of any homeopathic training.

Chakras and Corresponding Remedies
Here a few suggestions of polychrest homeopathic remedies and the chakras with which they have a particularly strong affinity. Obviously most remedies have an effect on more than one energy-centre, but it is still helpful to understand where the main emphasis of the remedy's action lies.

Chakra	Remedies
Crown	*Baryta-carb; Cannabis-indica; Hydrogen*
Brow	*Anhalonium; Luna; Medorrhinum*
Throat	*Iodum; Mercurius; Tuberculinum*
Heart	*Aurum; Ignatia; Natrum-mur; Lachesis*
Solar Plexus	*Arg.-nit.; Lycopodium; Nux-vomica; Phosphorus*
Sacral	*Lac-caninum; Sepia; Staphysagria; Thuja*
Base	*Arnica; Arsenicum; Gelsemium; Psorinum*

Case Examples

I have seen many cases where an awareness of the location of a disturbance within the chakra system enhanced my understanding of what needed treating and what kind of remedies might be helpful. Often I have noticed that during a consultation people will tend to protect the area of their energy body where they are vulnerable or where their energy is blocked, usually with their hands, folded arms, crossed legs or a similar unconscious gesture.

One patient I remember always clasped both hands tightly across her abdomen in the region of the solar plexus chakra. This immediately pointed to issues with self-confidence, fears and possibly anger. She had physical complaints of indigestion, flatulence and various food intolerances. The remedy that was clearly indicated on every level was *Lycopodium*, which I have come to realise is probably the leading polychrest with a solar-plexus chakra affinity.

One advantage of understanding the energy state of the chakras is that a cross-reference can be made between a person's physical and emotional state. I have seen many patients with chronic coughs which failed to clear up with well-indicated remedies. Knowing that the heart chakra (which relates to the whole chest area, including the lungs) is associated with grief and sadness, I have often found that *Ignatia* will cure these coughs even when it doesn't seem to match the symptoms exactly. Just as *Lycopodium* has an affinity with the solar-plexus chakra, so *Ignatia* has an affinity with the heart chakra, and can be prescribed by correspondence when indicated remedies fail to act.

On one occasion I prescribed *Medorrhinum* 30 to a patient suffering with chronic catarrh, sinus trouble and some joint problems. Immediately after taking it she had some profoundly vivid dreams, and then began to see the auras of people around her - something which had never happened before. This alerted to me the affinity that *Medorrhinum* has with the brow chakra, situated at the site of the 'third eye'. This chakra is associated with clairvoyant vision and the dream faculty, among other things. I have subsequently found that many people with sinus trouble and frontal headaches have congested energy in the brow chakra, which may be associated with a latent clairvoyant or other kind of psychic sensitivity.

I have found that understanding remedies according to their chakra affinities often helps to make sense of some of the strange symptoms that many remedies seem to have. For example, the base chakra is associated with survival issues, and is often blocked energetically when there is a history of violence, injury or abuse - i.e. any situation where a person has felt that their survival may be in danger. *Anacardium* is a remedy that is often indicated for someone with this kind of history, which would suggest that it has a base chakra affinity. Interestingly, one of the super-keynotes of *Anacardium* is a sensation as if the rectum were plugged up, which is a perfect physical description of an energy blockage in the base chakra! I imagine that as our understanding and knowledge of the human energy system grows, we will develop a correspondingly deeper understanding of our materia medica also.

Further Reading
A. Judith
Eastern Body, Western Mind
Wheels of Life
Celestial Arts, Berkeley, California

C. Myss
Anatomy of the Spirit
Bantam Books, London

C. Page
Frontiers of Health
C.W. Daniel Co., Saffron Walden, Essex

I. Watson
Health & The Planets
Homeopathy & the Chakras
Recorded Seminars, available in Audiotape and CD formats
www.ianwatsonseminars.com

Therapeutics

The fact is we need any and every way of finding the right remedy.

J. Compton-Burnett

Synonyms: Clinical Prescribing

Definition
Therapeutics means that a prescription is arrived at by differentiating between a group of remedies that are known to have a proven clinical relationship to a particular disease process.

Prescribing Technique
In therapeutics, the emphasis is on treating the disease process rather than treating the person. In common with other homeopathic techniques, however, therapeutics depends upon individualisation of each case of disease in order to be consistently effective. The basic technique involves taking as complete a case as possible of the disorder, for which purpose 'CLAMS' is a helpful tool (see Symptoms). Reference is then made either to a therapeutics book that includes the disease to be treated, or to a repertory and materia medica.

Usually several remedies will appear more or less well-indicated, and the outstanding and characteristic symptoms in the case must be used to differentiate between them. If there are marked concomitant symptoms to be found that relate to the general or mental state of the patient, these will often provide the differentiation between the group of remedies that cover the symptoms of the disease. With some practice, one learns to recognise the key symptoms in a case that will eliminate the majority of possible remedies and this narrows the analysis down to the relevant smaller group very quickly.

All of the major polychrest remedies have a range of therapeutic uses within their symptom pictures which allows them to be prescribed on a relatively small 'totality of symptoms'. As an example, I recently gave *Pulsatilla* to a man who had a cold which had gone onto his chest, with thick, yellow-green catarrh, more profuse in the morning. The remedy cleared up his condition almost immediately despite the fact that the constitutional remedy that had always helped him the most was *Phosphorus* rather than *Pulsatilla*. I have often heard students remark that a patient couldn't be given a certain remedy because it didn't fit their temperament or constitutional type, but it should be remembered that in a therapeutics situation it is the disorder that is to be treated rather than the constitution.

A homeopath who makes good use of therapeutics will also find opportunities to prescribe many of the smaller remedies in our materia medica which tend to be largely neglected in favour of the familiar polychrests.

Therapeutics Books

It will pay dividends for any student or practitioner to create their own alphabetical therapeutics book, which ideally should be a loose-leaf type book that can be easily updated without destroying the structure. The aim is to jot down the distinguishing symptoms of the most frequently prescribed remedies in the disorder concerned. It is far more useful to thoroughly learn the top six remedies say, for headaches, than to write out indications for every single remedy that appears in the *Repertory* under 'Headache', because the rubric contains many remedies that are very rarely needed in practice. It also makes sense to start out with the disorders that you are most likely to encounter on a regular basis, such as headaches, influenza, earaches, sore throats, etc., and to learn these thoroughly. Further disorders and additional remedies can be added as one's experience grows.

You find with experience that once you have treated a dozen or so sore throats using your own therapeutics book to help you, many of the essential features of the remedies listed will be retained in your mind and you will have to consult the book less and less frequently. This has the advantage of speeding up your prescribing considerably, and it also enables you to streamline your casetaking because you can eliminate and discriminate between remedies as you gather the information. I found that I also reached a point with disorders that I had treated regularly where I would know very quickly once the case had been taken whether the needed remedy was amongst my 'top six', or whether it was a less-frequently used remedy that was outside that group. As long as you are able to use therapeutics in a flexible way, amending and updating your groups of remedies according to your own experience, then the approach has many advantages.

Use of a Repertory

When a patient presents for treatment and the symptom-picture is unfamiliar then a repertory will often help in narrowing the selection down to a small group of remedies for comparison. Where the disease diagnosis is clear and unambiguous then the corresponding rubric in the repertory can be used as the starting point from which to eliminate further. Murphy's *Repertory* contains many disease rubrics showing those remedies that have a proven clinical record in each particular disease. Examples of such rubrics that I have found helpful in therapeutic practice include 'Angina pectoris' (p.1014), 'Emphysema' (p. 1215), 'Measles' (p. 708), 'Uterine fibroids' (p. 659) and 'Stomach ulcers' (p. 1770). It is worthwhile familiarising oneself with these clinical rubrics so that they may easily be located when they are needed.

When to Use Therapeutics

This method is useful in any situation where the nature of the disease process may be clearly ascertained, and it is the disease that is primarily to be treated. It can be an effective way of saving time and is therefore especially suited to the treatment of acute diseases and first-aid situations. However, chronic pathological states may also be treated successfully in this way.

Therapeutics is often the only prescribing technique (along with Specifics) that can be employed by general practitioners, pharmacists and others who are prescribing for large numbers of patients within very limited time constraints. Provided a degree of individualisation takes place, curative results can be obtained and many patients who would otherwise be given drugs can be helped with homeopathy. Because therapeutics emphasises the problem that the patient complains of, many people find they can relate to it very easily and it therefore provides an important bridge between allopathic medicine and constitutional homeopathy.

Case Examples

Case One

A woman, who had received constitutional treatment in the past and had responded extremely well, called to report a sudden attack of bursitis, affecting her left knee joint. It had swelled up enormously, was excruciatingly painful and she couldn't put her weight upon it. She felt almost faint with the pain. She had taken *Belladonna* and *Rhus tox.* already but neither remedy had helped. Her doctor had drawn a considerable quantity of fluid from the swelling but this failed to give any relief either. I questioned her carefully in order to clarify the remedy picture.

As far as could be ascertained, there was no obvious cause for the condition. The chief modality was that the pain was aggravated by lying with any weight on the leg - she said that the *pain seemed to travel to the part on which she lay.* She found that she could gain some relief by hanging her leg over the side of the bed, but after a while the *pain seemed to travel to the side which was*

122

hanging down.

The remedies *Bryonia, Apis, Ruta* and *Pulsatilla* were considered for this case. The aggravation from lying on the affected side ruled out *Bryonia*, and the absence stining pains and temperature modalities ruled out *Apis*. *Ruta* had the affinity for the problem area but the modalities were not to be found.

Considering the shifting, wandering pains and the aggravation from hanging the affected part down, I prescribed *Pulsatilla* 6 to be taken every two hours. Within a day the swelling had reduced considerably and the pain had almost disappeared. Over the next few days she recovered completely with a few more doses of the remedy.

Case Two

A woman had suffered for three weeks with frequent attacks of excruciating pain in the first three fingers of her right hand, and occasional tingling in the same fingers. She worked in a fish and chip shop and was using her right hand for lifting every day. The diagnosis was carpal tunnel syndrome, and she had been told that surgery was the only answer. Her general health was excellent.

This is an ideal case for a therapeutics approach because there are no general or constitutional symptoms on which to prescribe. It is therefore necessary to focus on the problem area itself and find a remedy which is similar to that. The factors to be considered then are firstly the *affinities* - fibrous tissues and nerves, suggesting *Rhus tox., Ruta, Hypericum* and *Bryonia* for consideration. Secondly the *nature* of the problem - compression of the nerve by the ligament, suggesting *Rhus tox* and *Ruta* particularly. Thirdly, the *likely causation* - overuse of the part, again suggesting *Rhus tox* and *Ruta* most strongly. There being no clear modalities of *Rhus tox* such as aggravation from first motion, *Ruta* seemed the overall best choice. *Ruta* is also known to have a stronger affinity for the ligaments and tendons than the other remedies considered.

On this basis she was given a dose of *Ruta* 50M, which cleared the condition completely within 24 hours. At the time of writing (approximately three years later) there has never been a return of the problem and her general health remains excellent.

Case Three

A woman presented with shingles across her rib-cage on the left side, of one week's duration. There were blisters which then formed into little scabs; itching, and a sharp, stabbing pain aggravated by movement. On consulting Tyler's

Pointers to the Common Remedies, Arsenicum, Mezereum, Ranunuculus-bulbosus and *Rhus-tox* was studied by comparison. the location was most characteristic of *Ranunuculus,* and the combiation of blisters, scabs and pain aggravated by movement were all covered by the remedy. she was consequently given three doses of *Ranunuculus-bulbosus* 10M and all of the symptoms had subsided within 48 hours.

Further Reading

Below are listed some of the more comprehensive therapeutics books, each of which give differentiations on many types of disorder. There are, in addition, hundreds of other works available each concentrating on a specific topic such as asthma, cancer, children's diseases, heart disease etc. The reader is advised to browse these before buying as there is a lot of duplication of material amongst them.

J. H. Clarke
The Prescriber
C. W. Daniel Co. Ltd., Saffron Walden, Essex

S. Lilienthal
Homeopathic Therapeutics
Jain Publishing Co., New Delhi, India

R. B. Bishamber Das
Select Your Remedy
Vishwamber Free Home Dispensary, New Delhi, India

J. N. Shinghal
Quick Bed-Side Prescriber
B. Jain Publishers Ltd, New Delhi

V. H. Merani
The Practitioner's Handbook of Homeopathy
Jain Publishing Co., New Delhi, India

M. L. Tyler
Pointers to the Common Remedies
The British Homeopathic Association, 27a Devonshire Street, London

W. A. Dewey
Practical Homeopathic Therapeutics
Jain Publishing Co., New Delhi, India

T. S. Hoyne
Clinical Therapeutics
Jain Publishing Co., New Delhi, India

E. A. Farrington
Clinical Materia Medica
Jain Publishing Co., New Delhi, India

R. Morrison
Desktop Companion to Physical Pathology
Hahnemann Clinic Publishing, Nevada City, U.S.A.

References

Aetiologies

1   J. T. Kent
   Repertory of the Homeopathic Materia Medica
   Jain Publishing Co., New Delhi, India

2   M. Tyler
   Homeopathic Drug Pictures
   C. W. Daniel Co. Ltd., Saffron Walden, Essex

3   H. C. Allen
   The Materia Medica of the Nosodes
   Jain Publishing Co., New Delhi, India

4   J. H. Clarke
   The Prescriber
   Health Science Press, C. W. Daniel Co. Ltd, Saffron Walden, Essex

Arborivital Medicine

1   R. T. Cooper
   Cancer and Cancer Symptoms, Chiefly Arborivital Treatment
   C. Marten, Wigmore Street, London; Second Edition, 1900

2   R. T. Cooper
   Arborivital Medicine: The Doctrine of Signatures from a Modern Point of View
   Homeopathic World, June 4, 1898, page 266

3   R. T. Cooper
   Cancer and Cancer Symptoms
   C. Marten, Wigmore Street, London; Second Edition, 1900

4   R. T. Cooper
   Cerebro-spinal Rhinorrhea
   Homeopathic World, November 1, 1899, page 489

Constitutional Prescribing

1   J. T. Kent
    Lectures on Homeopathic Philosophy
    Lesser Writings
    Jain Publishing Co., New Delhi, India

Genus Epidemicus

1   S. Hahnemann
    Organon of Medicine, 6th Edition, paras. 100-103
    Jain Publishing Co., New Delhi, India

2   H.C. Allen
    Materia Medica of the Nosodes
    Jain Publishing Co., New Delhi, India

3   J. T. Kent
    Lectures on Homeopathic Materia Medica, page 490
    Jain Publishing Co., New Delhi, India

4   M. L. Tyler
    Homeopathic Drug Pictures, page 695-696
    C. W. Daniel Co., Ltd., Saffron Walden, Essex

Intuitive Prescribing

1   The Homeopath
    Journal of The Society of Homeopaths, Letters to the Editor
    Issue No. 74

2   The Bailey Flower Essences
    7/8 Nelson Road, Ilkley, West Yorks., LS29 8HN

Isopathy

4 S. Hahnemann
   Organon of Medicine, Trans. from the 5th & 6th Edition by R. E. Dudgeon
   Jain Publishing Co., New Delhi, India

Miasmatic Prescribing

1 J.H. Clarke
   The Prescriber, page 54
   C.W. Daniel Co. Ltd., Saffron Walden, Essex

2 D.M Foubister
   Tutorials in Homeopathy
   Beaconsfield Publishers

3 Rima Handley
   A Homeopathic Love Story, Chapters 9 and 10
   North Atlantic Books, Berkeley, California, U.S.A.

4 Gurudas
   Flower Essences and Vibrational Healing
   Brotherhood of Life, Inc., Albuquerque, New Mexico, U.S.A.

5 H.L. Coulter
   AIDS and Syphilis - The Hidden Link
   North Atlantic Books, Berkeley, California, U.S.A.

Organ Remedies

1 K. P. Muzumdar
   *Transactions of the 32nd International Homeopathic Medical Congress,
   India, 1977*
   page 64

Physical Generals

1   J. T. Kent
How to Use the Repertory
Reprinted in front section of *Kent's Repertory of the Homeopathic Materia Medica*
Jain Publishing Co., New Delhi, India

Polypharmacy

1   Rima Handley
A Homeopathic Love Story
North Atlantic Books, Berkeley, California, U.S.A.

2   J. H. Clarke
Dictionary of Practical Materia Medica, page 1625
C. W. Daniel Co., Ltd., Saffron Walden, Essex

3   J. H. Clarke
The Prescriber, page 376
C. W. Daniel Co., Ltd., Saffron Walden, Essex

Symptom Similarity

1   S. Hahnemann
Organon of Medicine (6th Edn)
Jain Publishing Co., New Delhi, India

2   Ibid.
Paragraph 153

Tautopathy

1   H. L. Coulter
Homeopathic Science and Modern Medicine; page 60
North Atlantic Books, California, U.S.A.

– Notes–

– Notes–

CPSIA information can be obtained at www.ICGtesting.com
Printed in the USA
LVOW07s1736291114

416201LV00001B/195/P